THIS IS TRIVIA!

DO YOU REMEMBER THAT?

Exercise Your Mind, Expand Your Intelligence, and Improve Your Mental Capabilities While Having Fun.

Minnie Potter

TABLE OF CONTENTS

THE SURPRISING BENEFITS OF TRIVIA GAMES FOR OLDER ADULTS

As we get older, it becomes increasingly important to fortify not only our bodies, but also our minds. One easy and fun way to accomplish this is by playing trivia games. Trivia is loads of fun, and it comes with some brilliant mental and social benefits. For example, the universal thrill of correctly answering obscure questions in a friendly, competitive environment. (Winning doesn't hurt, either!)

Benefit # 1: Trivia is Fun!

Health and wellness benefits aside, trivia is a great activity for seniors for one very simple reason: It's fun!

According to health experts, trivia players experience a pleasant rush of dopamine when they know the answer to a question. This surge of feel-good chemicals in the brain is similar to what a person might feel while gambling. Unlike gambling, however, trivia doesn't come with any negative consequences like addiction or financial distress.

Even if your loved one is experiencing signs of dementia, they can excel at trivia games. For people with dementia, retrieving short-term memories can be difficult, whereas older memories are often recalled with great detail. So, while your loved one may have a hard time remembering what he or she ate for breakfast, they might easily recall which year Elvis Presley released Heartbreak Hotel was released (1956, FYI.)

Answering trivia questions can be extraordinarily validating for individuals who struggle with other everyday areas of life. It offers participants a boost of confidence and a sense of accomplishment, something most of us could use more of.

Benefit # 2: Trivia Enhances Memory

Your brain is a muscle, and just like the rest of the muscles in your body, it needs exercise to stay in tip-top shape. Think of trivia like a workout for your mind. It exercises the brain's frontal cortex, the part of the brain responsible for memory function. This, in turn, improves cognitive skills and problem-solving abilities.

Research shows that people who participate in mentally and socially stimulating activities enjoy greater cognitive function than those who don't. Delivering obscure facts about niche topics is an effective way to give your brain a boost while warding off the progression of age-related memory loss.

Trivia is as much about gaining new knowledge as it is about recalling old bits of information. Naturally, there will be questions that leave participants stumped. Learning the correct answers to these questions helps to keep our brains functioning optimally.

Benefit # 3: Trivia Reduces Stress

Getting older can be stressful, and if you're dealing with the effects of dementia, age-related stress can be cruelly compounded. Left unchecked, stress can wreak havoc on our health, so it's important to keep it under control. A fun game of trivia with friends can be the perfect antidote.

Getting together with friends in a relaxed environment is a great way to blow off steam and boost your happiness. Trivia encourages players to put down their phones for a couple of hours and just enjoy the moment. You really can't beat that.

Benefit # 4: Trivia Connects People

Of course, we can't overlook the social aspect of playing trivia games. For adults struggling with feelings of isolation, this is perhaps the most valuable element of trivia. Trivia offers participants a change of scene and the opportunity to socialize with friends. Playing on a team also gives people a valuable sense of community and camaraderie.

A bit of friendly competition can be beneficial as well. It encourages your loved one to challenge themself and try something new.

So, how about a little trivia? Have fun!

US & WORLD HISTORY

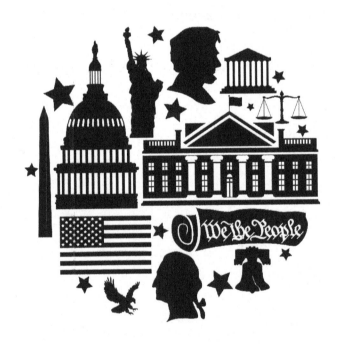

1. Who was the American Vice-President when the US entered the WWII war?

2. Who was the world heavyweight boxing champion for most of the 1940s?

3. This Hollywood gossip maven had a popular radio show and wrote an influential newspaper column for the LA Times for more than 20 years. She was at the zenith of her power in the 1940s and was known for wearing outlandish hats. Which woman was she?

4. When did President Franklin Roosevelt die?

5. According to the US Bureau of the Census which was NOT one of the five largest US cities in the 1940s?

6. This motorcycle organization was founded in Fontana, California in 1948. Rumor has it that its rules include that no prospective member may have ever applied to be in law enforcement. Can you name this rebel group?

7. In 1942, the U.S. Congress creates several branches of the armed forces for women to join the war effort. Can you name these branches?

8. What did the acronym "WAVES" stand for in the Navy's WAVES?

9. With the signing of the Treaty of Paris on December 10, 1898, Spain ceded these islands to the United States. And on July 4, 1946, the US formally recognized their independence, thus becoming the Republic of...?

10. In 1943, what building, considered to be the world's largest office building, was completed? Tip: It is located in Arlington, VA.

11. What agency was created when President Harry S. Truman signed the National Security Act of 1947 into law?

12. What new technology helped the British RAF (*Royal Air Force*) in defending against the Germans in WWII?

13. What was the Royal Air Force (RAF) called in World War I?

14. What was the popular name used for Operation Overlord during World War II in 1944?

15. On the same note, how did D-Day get its name?

16. What did the Kon-Tiki expedition set out to prove in 1947?

17. In 1942, the minimum draft age is lowered from 21 years old to what age in the United States?

18. In what country were the Lascaux prehistoric cave paintings discovered in 1940?

19. In 1940 which world leader made the speeches "We Shall Fight Them On The Beaches....." and "Never in the field of human conflict was so much..." ?

20. What is the name of the radio broadcasting network of the U.S. government that began service in 1942? Why was it created?

21. What was the Warsaw Jewish Ghetto uprising against the Nazis in 1943?

22. In what year was an UFO allegedly found on July 7th in the Roswell UFO incident?

23. In 1949, NATO was established, what does NATO stand for?

24. In what year did The United Nations vote in favor for the creation of an Independent Jewish State of Israel?

25. During World War II, US Gas Rationing allowed how many gallons of gas per week in 1942?

26. What did the Fair Labor Standards Act of 1938 accomplish?

27. During World War II, what did Executive Order 9066 do in 1942?

28. In 1949, the Communist People's Republic of China is proclaimed under which leader?

29. What city was the site of the 900-Day Siege during World War II?

30. In 1943, due to shortages in copper in the U.S., the one-cent coin is struck in what metal during World War II?

31. In what year Germany invade Denmark, Norway, France, Luxembourg, Belgium, and Netherlands?

32. In 1941, U.S. President Franklin D. Roosevelt signed what bill to provide financial aid to veterans who returned from World War II?

33. What was The Marshall Plan signed in 1948 about? Which president signed it?

34. In what year was Apartheid made the official policy of the National Party in South Africa?

35. When did Apartheid end as an official policy in South Africa?

36. Why did the USS Indianapolis, a *Portland-class heavy cruiser, sank on July 30, 1945?*

37. Who was the "Little Boy"?

38. Who was Enola Gay?

39. Which president remains the only president to have served for more than two terms? He served four terms.

40. What does the 22nd amendment passed on by Congress in 1947 say and why was it passed?

41. On the same note, how many terms did George Washington serve and why?

42. Name the allegorical cultural icon in the United States who represents the women who worked in factories and shipyards during World War II.

43. Who was Canada's equivalent of Rosie the Riveter?

44. Who invented the "Aqua-Lung"?

45. Which legendary band leader disappeared whilst on board a military plane in 1944 while on his way to perform for the troops in Paris for Christmas?

46. What terrible events took place on August 6th and August 9th, 1945?

47. What is the codename for the secret US government research and engineering project during the Second World War that developed the world's first nuclear weapons?

48. On October 24, 1946, the first ever picture from outer space of which plant was taken?

49. Who are the four heads carved in Mount Rushmore?

50. Red Baron is a household name, even for non-aviation fans. Why did he achieve such fame?

ANSWERS 1 - 50
US & WORLD HISTORY

1. Henry Wallace

The US declared war on Japan immediately following the bombing of Pearl Harbor on December 7, 1941, and war with Germany and Italy followed within a few days. Henry Wallace had succeeded John Nance Garner as vice-president in January 1941. He was replaced on the 1944 Democratic ticket by Missouri Senator Harry Truman because party leaders feared for President Roosevelt's health and felt Truman was a more neutral choice should he succeed Roosevelt as president.

2. Joe Louis

Joe Louis ruled the heavyweight ring from 1937 to mid-1949.

World War II raged early in the decade, and just like baseballers, many popular boxers went overseas to fight for their countries, Joe Louis, Billy Conn, Beau Jack, and Bob Montgomery among them. Louis was used to entice Americans to join the war against Germany, a couple of propaganda movies starring Louis and many propaganda posters being produced. The posters are collectors' items today.

Louis' great rival, Max Schmeling, a lifelong opponent of the Nazi regime, was forced by Adolf Hitler to join the German military after his loss to Louis at their 1938 rematch

3. Hedda Hopper

Hopper's son, William Hopper, played private detective Paul Drake on the "Perry Mason" television show (1957-1966). Louella Parsons was a rival columnist and the founder of the Hollywood Women's Press Club.

4. April 12, 1945.

He had been inaugurated on January 20th for his fourth term as president, an unprecedented feat never to be repeated. He was only 63 years old, but his health had been undermined with many conditions, very high blood pressure, congestive heart failure, possibly melanoma, that today might have been ameliorated with medication.

He was weakened by post-polio syndrome and the enormous stresses of 12 years of overseeing the nation's recovery from the Great Depression and heading up the wartime coalition to defeat the Germans, Japanese and their allies.

5. Boston

Boston was ranked the 9th largest US city in the 1940s. New York was #1, Chicago was #2, Philadelphia was #3, Detroit was #4 and Los Angeles was #5. Times change - by 1990, Boston had dropped to the #20.

6. Hell's Angels

The Hells Angels originated on March 17, 1948, in Fontana, California, when several small motorcycle clubs agreed to merge. Otto Friedli, a World War II veteran, is credited with starting the club.

To become a Hell's Angels prospect, candidates must have a valid driver's license, a motorcycle over 750cc, and the right combination of personal qualities.

7. The Army's Women's Auxiliary Corps or WACs, the Navy's WAVES, the Coast Guard's SPARs, and the Women Air Force Service Pilots.

Several hundred thousand women volunteered to "free a man to fight." They were issued uniforms and replaced soldiers in clerical and other non-combat related jobs. Women were restricted from combat zones; however, many became nurses to help the men injured in combat.

8. Women Accepted for Volunteer Emergency Service

Members of the WAVES worked in fields ranging from secretarial and clerical duties to jobs in the aviation, intelligence, medical and communications communities.

9. The Republic of the Philippines

In 1935, the Commonwealth of the Philippines was established with U.S. approval, and Manuel Quezon was elected the country's first president. On July 4, 1946, full independence was granted to the Republic of the Philippines by the United States.

10. The Pentagon

At its completion at a cost of $83 million in January 1943, the Pentagon was the world's largest office building, covering 29 acres (12 hectares) including a 5-acre (2-hectare) central court and containing roughly 3,700,000 square feet (344,000 square meters) of usable floor space for approximately 25,000 people.

11. The United States Central Intelligence Agency (CIA)

A major impetus that has been cited over the years for the creation of the CIA was the unforeseen attack on Pearl Harbor, but whatever Pearl Harbor's role, in the twilight of World War II it was considered clear in government circles that there was a need for a group to coordinate government intelligence efforts, and the Federal Bureau of Investigation (FBI), the State

Department, and the War Department, and even the Post Office were all jockeying for that new power.

12. Radar or radio detecting and ranging

It was one of the most important factors in the success of Britain's air defenses during the Battle of Britain.
Radar could be used to detect and locate incoming enemy aircraft. It worked by sending out radio waves which would bounce off solid objects at a distance, enabling operators to estimate four important things about approaching raids: the range (distance), bearing (direction), strength and height.

13. The Royal Flying Corps (RFC)

They were the air arm of the British Army before and during the First World War until it merged with the Royal Naval Air Service on 1 April 1918 to form the Royal Air Force.

14. D-Day, The landing of Allied troops in Normandy, France.

Allied forces launched the largest amphibious invasion in the history of warfare. Codenamed Operation 'Overlord', the Allied landings on the beaches of Normandy marked the start of a long and costly campaign to liberate north-west Europe from Nazi occupation.

15. According to the U.S. military, "D-Day" was an Army designation used to indicate the start date for specific field operations.

In this case, the "D" in D-Day doesn't actually stand for anything—it's merely an alliterative placeholder used to designate a particular day on the calendar.

16. In the Voyage of the Kon-Tiki, it was proved that early humans could have used the trade winds to sail from Peru to Easter Island - and thus be its first settlers.

On August 7, 1947, *Kon-Tiki*, a balsa wood raft captained by Norwegian anthropologist Thor Heyerdahl, completes a 4,300-mile, 101-day journey from Peru to Raroia in the Tuamotu Archipelago, near Tahiti.

Heyerdahl and his five-person crew set sail from Callao, Peru, on the 45-foot-long *Kon-Tiki* on April 28, 1947. The *Kon-Tiki*, named for a mythical white chieftain, was made of indigenous materials and designed to resemble rafts of early South American Indians. While crossing the Pacific, the sailors encountered storms, sharks and whales, before finally washing ashore at Raroia.

17. 18 years old

On November 11, 1942, Congress approves lowering the draft age to 18 and raising he upper limit to age 37.

-In September 1940, Congress, by wide margins in both houses, passed the Burke-Wadsworth Act, and the first peacetime draft was imposed in the history of the United States

18. France

Near Montignac, France, a collection of prehistoric cave paintings are discovered by four teenagers who stumbled upon the ancient artwork after following their dog down a narrow entrance into a cavern.

19. Winston Churchill

The summer of 1940 saw the Battle of Britain, the aerial conflict between the Royal Air Force and the German Luftwaffere, reach its apex. When in this speech Churchill stated, 'Never in the field of human conflict was so much been owed by so many to so few', he was paying tribute to the enormous efforts made by the fighter pilots and bomber crews to establish air superiority over England.

20. Voice of America (VOA)

Its first broadcast, in German, took place on February 24, 1942, and was intended to counter Nazi propaganda among the German people. By the time World War II ended, the VOA was broadcasting 3,200 programs in 40 languages every week. It became part of the USIA when that agency was established in 1953.

Ever since its birth, the VOA has served the world with a consistent message of truth, hope and inspiration.

21. The Warsaw Ghetto Uprising was an act of Jewish resistance in the Warsaw Ghetto in German-occupied Poland during World War II to oppose Nazi Germany's final effort to transport the remaining ghetto population to Majdanek and Treblinka death camps.

The uprising started on 19 April when the ghetto refused to surrender to the police commander SS-Brigadeführer Jürgen Stroop, who ordered the burning of the ghetto, block by block, ending on 16 May. The uprising was the largest single revolt by Jews during World War II.

22. 1947

23. North Atlantic Treaty Organization

The North Atlantic Alliance was founded in the aftermath of the Second World War. Its purpose was to secure peace in Europe, to promote cooperation among its members and to guard their freedom – all of this in the context of countering the threat posed at the time by the Soviet Union.

24. 1947

On 29 November 1947, a 2000-year-old dream became reality: A Jewish State was born anew in its ancient homeland. On that day the UN General Assembly voted on Resolution 181, adopting a plan to partition the British Mandate into two states, one Jewish, one Arab.

25. 4 Gallons

By December of 1942, rubber and gasoline were added to the list of rationed items. The OPA issued stickers, which were placed on your windshield, to determine how much gasoline you were entitled to. The "A" sticker was the most common and entitled you to four gallons a week.

In addition to rationing gasoline, the speed limit was established at 35 MPH for the duration of the war. The rationing of gas was done not only to conserve gasoline but also to conserve tires.

26. It limited the workweek in the US to 44 hours.

This act was amended on June 26, 1940, to reduce the workweek to 40 hours, therefore, the 40-hour workweek became U.S. law.

The Fair Labor Standards Act (FLSA) establishes minimum wage, overtime pay, recordkeeping, and youth employment standards affecting employees in the private sector and in Federal, State, and local governments.

27. Allowed Japanese Americans to be put into internment camps.

Issued by President Franklin Roosevelt on February 19, 1942, this order authorized the evacuation of all persons deemed a threat to national security from the West Coast to relocation centers further inland. In the next 6 months, over 100,000 men, women, and children of Japanese ancestry were moved to assembly centers.

28. Mao Zedong or *Mao Tse-tung*

Mao Zedong (26 December 1893 – 9 September 1976), also known as Chairman Mao, was a Chinese communist revolutionary who was the founder of the People's Republic of China (PRC), which he led as the chairman of the Chinese Communist Party from the establishment of the PRC in 1949 until his death in 1976.

29. Leningrad, encircled by the German Army Group North, never fell, despite the long siege.

The siege of Leningrad, also known as the 900-Day Siege though it lasted a grueling 872 days, resulted in the deaths of some one million of the city's civilians and Red Army defenders. Leningrad, formerly St. Petersburg, capital of the Russian Empire, was one of the initial targets of the German invasion of June 1941.

30. Steel

The 1943 steel cent, also known as a steel war penny or steelie, was a variety of the U.S. one-cent coin which was struck in steel due to wartime shortages of copper, which was needed for ammunition and other military equipment during World War II.

31. 1940

Using the Blitzkrieg tactic, Germany defeated Poland, Denmark, Norway, Belgium, the Netherlands, Luxembourg, France, Yugoslavia, and Greece. Yet Germany did not defeat Great Britain, which was protected from ground attack by the English Channel.

32. G.I. Bill

Officially the Servicemen's Readjustment Act of 1944, the G.I. Bill was created to help veterans of World War II. From 1944 to 1949, nearly 9 million veterans received close to $4 billion from the bill's unemployment compensation program.

33. It was signed by President Truman. It was an agreement that allowed the US to send over $13 billion in aid to Europe between 1948 and 1951.

On April 3, 1948, President Truman signed the Economic Recovery Act of 1948. It became known as the Marshall Plan, named for Secretary of State George Marshall, who in 1947 proposed that the United States provide economic assistance to restore the economic infrastructure of postwar Europe.

34. 1948

Beginning in 1948 following the general election, the party as the governing party of South Africa began implementing its policy of racial segregation, known as apartheid (the Afrikaans term for "separateness").

35. It came to an end in the early 1990s in a series of steps that led to the formation of a democratic government in 1994.

Under the administration of the South African president F.W. de Klerk, legislation supporting apartheid was repealed in the early 1990s, and a new constitution, one that enfranchised blacks and other racial groups, was adopted in 1993.

All-race national elections held in 1994 resulted in a black majority government led by prominent anti-apartheid activist Nelson Mandela of the African National Congress party. Although these developments marked the end of legislated apartheid, the social and economic effects of apartheid remained deeply entrenched in South African society.

36. The USS Indianapolis is torpedoed by a Japanese submarine and sinks within minutes in shark-infested waters. Only 316 of the 1,196 men on board survived.

In July 1945, the USS Indianapolis completed a top-secret high-speed trip to deliver uranium and other components for "Little Boy" to the Tinian Naval Base, and subsequently departed for the Philippines on training duty.

It sank in 12 minutes. Of 1,195 crewmen aboard, approximately 300 went down with the ship. The remaining 890 faced exposure, dehydration, saltwater poisoning, and shark attacks while stranded in the open ocean with few lifeboats and almost no food or water. The Navy only learned of the sinking four days later and only 316 men survived.

37. The atomic bomb used at Hiroshima, Japan, on August 6, 1945. It was the first nuclear weapon used in warfare.

The bomb weighed 9,000 pounds and had a diameter of only 28 inches. The gun-type weapon possessed the power of 26,000,000 pounds of high explosives. Little Boy was dropped untested.

Previously, on July 26, the bomb, along with "Fat Man", another bomb, had been transported to Tinian Island by USS Indianapolis for final assembly. Four days later, Japanese submarine, I-58, sank Indianapolis, northeast of Leyte.

38. It was the B-29 bomber that was used by the United States on August 6, 1945, to drop "Little Boy", the first atomic bomb on Hiroshima, Japan.

The aircraft was named after the mother of its pilot Paul Warfield Tibbets, Jr. It became the first aircraft to drop an atomic bomb in warfare.

39. Franklin D. Roosevelt

The third presidential term of Franklin D. Roosevelt began on January 20, 1941, when he was once again inaugurated as the 32nd president of the United States, and the fourth term of his presidency ended with his death on April 12, 1945, on year after he had been re-elected.

Unlike his first two terms, Roosevelt's third and fourth terms were dominated by foreign policy concerns, as the United States became involved in World War II in December 1941.

40. Passed by Congress in 1947, and ratified by the states on February 27, 1951, the Twenty-Second Amendment limits an elected president to two terms in office, a total of eight years. However, it is possible for an individual to serve up to ten years as president.

41. He served only two terms.

Mindful of the precedent his conduct set for future presidents, Washington feared that if he were to die while in office, Americans would view the presidency as a lifetime appointment. Instead, he decided to step down from power, providing the standard of a two-term limit.

42. Rosie the Riveter

Many of these women produced munitions and war supplies and would sometimes take entirely new jobs replacing the male workers who joined the military. Rosie the Riveter is used as a symbol of American feminism and women's economic advantage
Similar images of women war workers appeared in other countries such as Britain and Australia.

The idea of Rosie the Riveter originated in a song written in 1942 by Redd Evans and John Jacob Loeb. Images of women workers were widespread in the media in formats such as government posters, and commercial advertising was heavily used by the government to encourage women to volunteer for wartime service in factories.

43. Veronica Foster (January 2, 1922 – May 4, 2000), popularly known as "Ronnie, the Bren Gun Girl".

Foster worked for John Inglis Company Ltd. Producing Bren light machine guns on a production line on Strachan Avenue in Toronto, Ontario. While working at the John Inglis Company Ltd. she was photographed for a propaganda campaign to encourage Canadian women to participate in the war efforts. She can be seen as the Canadian precursor to Rosie the Riveter.

44. French naval officer Jacques-Yves Cousteau and Air Liquide engineer Emile Gagnan.

In 1943 they developed an autonomous diving system with a demand regulator, the scaphandre autonome. It would soon be called "Aqua-Lung," after Cousteau coined the word for English-speaking countries.

45. Glen Miller

The news broke most places on Christmas Day 1944, crammed onto front pages amid the blaring war headlines: Glenn Miller was missing. The legendary American big band leader, whose music cheered the war-weary and thrilled a generation, had vanished over the English Channel while flying from Britain to France.

The wreckage of Miller's plane was never found. His official military status remains Missing in Action.

46. On August 6, 1945, the United States dropped an atomic bomb on the city of Hiroshima. The bomb was known as "Little Boy", a uranium gun-type bomb that exploded with about thirteen kilotons of force.

Three days after the United States dropped an atomic bomb on Hiroshima, a second atomic bomb was dropped on Nagasaki on August 9 – a 21-kiloton plutonium device known as "Fat Man.

First and foremost, the bombs were dropped to bring the war with Japan to a speedy end and spare American lives. It has been suggested that the second objective was to demonstrate the new weapon of mass destruction to the Soviet Union.

On August 14, Japan surrendered. Journalist George Weller was the "first into Nagasaki" and described the mysterious "atomic illness" (the onset of radiation sickness) that was killing patients who outwardly appeared to have escaped the bomb's impact.

The debate over the bomb, whether there should have been a test demonstration, whether the Nagasaki bomb was necessary, and more, continues to this day.

47. The Manhattan Project

It was led by the United States with the support of the United Kingdom and Canada. The Manhattan Project produced the first atomic bomb. The weapons produced were based solely upon the principles of nuclear fission of uranium 235 and plutonium 239, chain reactions liberating immense amounts of destructive heat energy. Eventually 130,000 people participated in the Manhattan Project. By July 1945, scientists had developed three atomic bombs.

President Franklin Roosevelt created a committee to look into the possibility of developing a nuclear weapon after he received a letter from Nobel Prize laureate Albert Einstein in October 1939. In his letter, Einstein warned the president that Nazi Germany was likely already at work on developing a nuclear weapon. By August 1942, the Manhattan Project was underway.

48. Planet Earth

It was taken with a camera installed on a rocket that launched from White Sands Missile Range, New Mexico.

The rocket was actually a Nazi V-2 ballistic missile prepared by a group of surrendered German rocket scientists. It flew to an altitude of about 65 miles (104 km) which is the agreed border of the outer space and took a series of pictures. The camera was enclosed in a steel case for protection as a few minutes later the camera hit the ground with an incredible speed.

49.
- **George Washington, First President of the United States**
- **Thomas Jefferson, Third President of the United States**
- **Theodore Roosevelt, 26th President of the United States**
- **Abraham Lincoln, 16th President of the United States.**

Did you know plan A for Mount Rushmore was to spotlight another set of four heads?

Believe it or not, Plan A was to spotlight regional heroes such as Lewis and Clark, Buffalo Bill Cody, and the Oglala Lakota leader, Red Cloud. The figures would be carved into the granite pillars known as The Needles. This, essentially, would have made the work similar to a set of totem poles.

50. The Red Baron was the name applied to Manfred von Richthofen, a German fighter pilot who was the deadliest flying ace of World War I.

Wonder where his name is coming from? His three-winged Fokker was painted in bright red so he would scare his enemies once they spotted him. He trained and flew with a unit called "The Flying Circus", by far the most feared by Allied forces. The Red Baron was finally shot and injured, but still managed to land his plane before he died.

51. Who was the first pilot to break the sound barrier in 1947?

52. James Doolittle organized one of the most daring mission strikes in WWII. Which one was it?

53. Which intergovernmental organization was founded on June 26, 1945, in San Francisco, CA?

54. What famous speech given by Sir Winston Churchill lead the way to the Cold War?

55. What is the Clean Air Act of 1956 signed in the UK? What led to its creation?

56. What was the name of Russia's first artificial satellite that was launched in 1957?

57. Who accompanied Sir Edmund Hillary as the first person to successfully climb the summit of Mount Everest in 1953?

58. Which country's lunar probe became the first man-made object to hit the moon in 1959?

59. Which Soviet leader became the Premier of the Soviet Union in 1958 after Georgi Malenkov, who succeeded Stalin in 1953?

60. In 1957 the British colony of the Gold Coast became the independent nation of ..?

61. What year did China invade Tibet?

62. Which Communist leader came to power after the Cuban Revolution in 1959?

63. Which popular entertainer was inducted into the US army in 1958?

64. Who were the Little Rock Nine and what did they do?

65. What did President Eisenhower do when Arkansas governor, Orval Faubus, ordered the National Guard to prevent the Little Rock Nine from entering the premises?

66. Which American civil rights leader refused to give up her seat in 1955?

67. What year did North Korea invade South Korea capturing Seoul?

68. What year did Puerto Rico become a self-governing commonwealth of the United States?

69. In 1957, Britain tested its first hydrogen bomb on what island?

70. Jack Kilby invented which important piece of technology in 1958? Tip: It led to the creation of cell phones and computers.

71. Which Wisconsin Senator was censured in 1954 after his seeking out Communists in the US government?

72. In what year were the words "Under God" added to the USA Pledge of Allegiance?

73. Which royal became Britain's head of state in 1953?

74. Which landmark Supreme Court case ended racial segregation in public schools in 1954?

75. Who discovered the "Double-Helix" structure of DNA in 1953?

76. Who is credited for developing the first Polio vaccine in 1953?

77. Which Japanese car manufacturer started selling cars in the USA in 1957?

78. In 1952, the Mau Mau Rebellion began in what country?

79. The nationalization of which canal led Israel, Britain, and France to attack Egypt in 1956?

80. Name the site that opened in 1892 at the mouth of the Hudson River as an immigration station, a purpose it served for more than 60 years until it closed in 1954.

81. On the same note, where did the name Ellis Island originate?

82. Under which president "In God We Trust", the current official US motto, was adopted?

83. On the same note, which was the previous official US motto?

84. What did The Federal Aid Highway Act of 1956 allow when it became a law?

85. Which agency was created when Eisenhower signed the National Aeronautics and Space Act in July 1958?

86. Which were the last two states to join the US?

87. On the same note, who sold Alaska to the US and for how much?

88. And, who owned the Hawaiian Islands before US?

89. On July 11, 1955, Congress passed H.R. 619 which mandated what to be included on all U.S. currency.

90. On the same note, when was the phrase "In God We Trust" stamped on US coins?

91. Who were the "Mercury Seven"?

92. What was built in Germany in 1961 that would symbolize the lack of freedom under communism?

93. Which independent agency and program of the United States government that trains and deploys volunteers to provide international development assistance was created by President John F. Kennedy on March 1, 1961?

94. Who was the first black student to enroll in the University of Mississippi?

95. What happened November 22, 1963, at 12:30 p.m. CST in Dallas, Texas?

96. On July 1, 1963, the Post Office Department introduced a plan to allow mail sorting methods to become faster and eventually automated. What is the name of that plan?

97. In 1965, the Gemini Mission astronauts brought along a drink mix brand. Do you remember the brand?

98. On the same note, do you recall which department store brand manufactured the US flag placed on the moon?

99. Which action by President Lyndon B. Johnson legally ended the segregation that had been institutionalized by Jim Crow laws?

100. On July 14, 1965, the first photos humans had ever seen of another world were taken. What was the name of the probe and the planet?

51. Brigadier General Charles Elwood Yeager

He became a famous pilot due to his audacity by breaking the sound barrier in 1947, in a Bell X-1. Yeager is still alive and recently broke the sound barrier again, in an F-15, to mark the 65th anniversary of the first supersonic flight.

52. The Doolittle Raid, also known as the Tokyo Raid, was an air raid on 18 April 1942 by the United States on the Japanese capital Tokyo and other places on Honshu during World War II. It was the first air operation to strike the Japanese archipelago.

It was to strike back after the Japanese attack on Pearl Harbor, but also the first attack on mainland Japan, an important psychological raid, to show the Japanese that they could be attacked. Doolittle organized the strike, known from the Movie "Pearl Harbor". It was an important US propaganda victory even though Doolittle himself saw it as a failure because of the losses.

53. The United Nations

As World War II was about to end in 1945, nations were in ruins, and the world wanted peace. Representatives of 50 countries gathered at the United Nations Conference on International Organization in San Francisco, California from 25 April to 26 June 1945.

For the next two months, they proceeded to draft and then sign the UN Charter, which created a new international organization, the United Nations, which, it was hoped, would prevent another world war like the one they had just lived through.

54. The "Iron Curtain" speech

On March 5, 1946, Sir Winston Churchill visited Westminster College as the Green Lecturer and delivered "Sinews of Peace," a message heard round the world that went down in history as the "Iron Curtain Speech."

The "Iron Curtain" term referred to the political, military, and ideological barrier erected by the Soviet Union after World War II to seal off itself and its dependent eastern and central European allies from open contact with the West and other noncommunist areas.

Stalin compared Churchill to Hitler and described him as "a warmonger" who aimed at "Anglo-Saxon ...racial" world domination. At the same time, he claimed that the Soviet Union, despite recent war losses, was capable of waging and winning another war.

55. The Clean Air Act was a regulation passed by the UK government to restrict the burning of coal in urban areas in the United Kingdom.

The Great Smog of London, or Great Smog of 1952, led to its establishment.

The Great Smog was a severe air pollution event that affected London, England, in December 1952.

During a cold snap on December 5th, sulphur particles mixed with fumes from burning coal and made the yellow fog smell like rotten eggs. Some Londoners reported being unable to see their feet, and transportation was canceled with the exception of the London Underground. Birds flew into buildings, and robberies increased as thieves were able to make an easy getaway.

The smog eventually lifted on December 9 after cold winds swept the fumes out to the North Sea.

56. Sputnik 1

History changed on October 4, 1957, when the Soviet Union successfully launched Sputnik I. The world's first artificial satellite was about the size of a beach ball (58 cm. or 22.8 inches in diameter), weighed only 83.6 kg. or 183.9 pounds and took about 98 minutes to orbit Earth on its elliptical path.

57. Sherpa Tenzing Norgay

At 11:30 a.m. on May 29, 1953, Edmund Hillary of New Zealand and Tenzing Norgay, a Sherpa of Nepal, become the first explorers to reach the summit of Mount Everest, which at 29,035 feet above sea level is the highest point on earth.

58. USSR (Soviet Union)

Prove Luna 9 launched on 31 January 1966 from Baikonur Cosmodrome and reached the Moon on 3 February. This prove became the first spacecraft to achieve a survivable landing on a celestial body.

When assembled, the photographs provided four panoramic views of the nearby lunar surface. Luna 9 survived three Earth-days on the surface until its batteries ran down. From the pictures, scientists could tell that the spacecraft had landed near an 82-foot (25-meter) crater.

59. Nikita Khrushchev

In 1956, Khrushchev (as First Secretary of the Central Committee of the Communist Party) made a secret speech to the congress condemning Stalin's regime and dictatorial rule. Shortly thereafter, he began to implement a series of reforms known as the thaw.

These reforms included transforming Soviet foreign policy to that of "peaceful cooperation" with the West and destroying the GULAG system and releasing thousands of political prisoners who had been incarcerated under Stalin. "Destalinization" continued after Khrushchev became prime minister in 1958.

60. Ghana

The Gold Coast was a British Crown colony on the Gulf of Guinea in West Africa from 1821 until its independence in 1957 as Ghana.

The first European explorers to arrive at the coast were the Portuguese in 1471. They encountered a variety of African kingdoms, some of which controlled substantial deposits of gold in the soil.

The Gold Coast had long been a name for the region used by Europeans because of the large gold resources found in the area. The slave trade was the principal exchange and major part of the economy for many years.

61. 1950

Tibet came under the control of People's Republic of China (PRC) after the Government of Tibet accepted the Seventeen Point Agreement under Chinese pressure in October 1951. This occurred after attempts by the Tibetan Government to gain international recognition, efforts to modernize its military, negotiations between the Government of Tibet and the PRC, and a military conflict in the Chamdo area of western Kham in October 1950

62. Fidel Castro

After Batista's overthrow in 1959, Castro assumed military and political power as Cuba's prime minister. The United States came to oppose Castro's government and unsuccessfully attempted to remove him by assassination, economic embargo, and counter-revolution, including the Bay of Pigs Invasion of 1961.

63. Elvis Presley

Elvis Presley as a US Soldier Stationed in West Germany: 1958-1960. When Elvis Presley walked off an army troop ship in Bremerhaven, West Germany on October 1, 1958, he was only 23 years old.

64. The Little Rock Nine were a group of nine African American students enrolled in Little Rock Central High School in 1957.

Their enrollment was followed by the Little Rock Crisis, in which the students were initially prevented from entering the racially segregated school by Orval Faubus, the Governor of Arkansas.

The Little Rock Nine are Ernest Green, Minnijean Brown, Elizabeth Eckford, Thelma Mothershed, Melba Pattillo, Gloria Ray, Terrence Roberts, Jefferson Thomas, and Carlotta Walls. In 1957 they were just teenagers, ranging in age from 15-17, but they were already among the bravest Arkansans.

65. President Eisenhower ordered the 101st Airborne Division into Little Rock to ensure the safety of the "Little Rock Nine" and that the rulings of the Supreme Court were upheld.

66. Rosa Parks

In 1955, Parks rejected a bus driver's order to leave a row of four seats in the "colored" section once the white section had filled up and move to the back of the bus. Her defiance sparked a successful boycott of buses in Montgomery a few days later. Residents refused to board the city's buses.

She helped initiate the civil rights movement in the United States when she refused to give up her seat to a white man on a Montgomery, Alabama bus in 1955.

67. 1950

The United States supported the South, the Soviet Union supported the North, and each government claimed sovereignty over the whole Korean peninsula. In 1950, after years of mutual hostilities, North Korea invaded South Korea in an attempt to re-unify the peninsula under its communist rule.

America wanted not just to contain communism, they also wanted to prevent the domino effect. Truman was worried that if Korea fell, the next country to fall would be Japan, which was very important for American trade. This was probably the most important reason for America's involvement in the war.

68. 1952

In 1951 Puerto Ricans overwhelmingly approved the commonwealth status in a referendum, and the island's constitution was proclaimed on July 25, 1952, a symbolic date because it was the 54th anniversary of the U.S. invasion of the island.

69. Christmas Island

Operation Grapple was a set of four series of British nuclear weapons tests of early atomic bombs and hydrogen bombs carried out in 1957 and 1958 at Malden Island and Kiritimati (Christmas Island) in the Gilbert and Ellice Islands in the Pacific Ocean (modern Kiribati)

70. The microchip

An American engineer, Jack Kilby, invented the integrated circuit – the microchip - in 1958, shortly after he began working at Texas Instruments. It would revolutionize the electronics industry, helping make cell phones and computers widespread today.

71. Joseph McCarthy

In 1954 McCarthy's investigation of security threats in the U.S. Army was televised. McCarthy's bullying of witnesses turned public opinion against the Senator. On December 2, 1954, the Senate voted to censure him, describing his behavior as "contrary to senatorial traditions."

72. 1954

The first version of the Pledge of Allegiance, which contained no reference to religion, was written for the Columbian Exposition in October 1892 to mark the 400th anniversary of Christopher Columbus' arrival in the Americas.

On June 14, 1954, President Dwight Eisenhower signed a bill to insert the phrase "under God" into the U.S. Pledge of Allegiance that children recited every morning in school.

The push to add "under God" to the pledge gained momentum during the second Red Scare, a period when U.S. politicians were keen to assert the moral superiority of U.S. capitalism over Soviet communism, which many conservatives regarded as "godless."

73. Queen Elizabeth II

The coronation of Elizabeth II took place on 2 June 1953 at Westminster Abbey in London. She acceded to the throne at the age of 25 upon the death of her father, George VI, on 6 February 1952, being proclaimed queen by her privy and executive councils shortly afterwards.

74. Brown v. Board of Education

Oliver Brown v. Board of Education of Topeka was a landmark 1954 Supreme Court case in which the justices ruled unanimously that racial segregation of children in public schools was unconstitutional.

75. James Watson and Francis Crick

These two young scientists declared to patrons of the Eagle Pub in Cambridge, England, that they had "found the secret of life." Their claim was a valid one, for they had in fact discovered the structure of DNA. The stunning find made possible the era of "new biology" that led to the biotechnology industry and, most recently, the deciphering of the human genetic blueprint.

76. Jonas Salk

On March 26, 1953, American medical researcher Dr. Jonas Salk announces on a national radio show that he tested his experimental killed-virus vaccine on himself and his family in 1953

77. Toyota

Toyota USA opened its doors on October 31, 1957. In its first full year of sales, the division sold 288 vehicles total: 287 Toyopet Crowns, and one Land Cruiser. The company almost gave up the US market, but persevered. Today, it's built 25 million cars in the US.

78. Kenya

The Mau Mau rebellion (1952–1960), also known as the Mau Mau uprising, Mau Mau revoltor Kenya Emergency, was a war in the British Kenya Colony (1920–1963) between the Kenya Land and Freedom Army (KLFA), also known as the Mau Mau, and the British authorities.

79. Suez Canal

Its value to international trade made it a nearly instant source of conflict among Egypt's neighbors and Cold War superpowers vying for dominance. The catalyst for the joint Israeli-British-French attack on Egypt was the nationalization of the Suez Canal by Egyptian leader Gamal Abdel Nasser in July 1956.

80. Ellis Island

Between 1892 and 1954, more than 12 million immigrants passed through Ellis Island in order to start a new life in the United States. They came to escape religious persecution, political oppression, and poverty in their home countries. Getting through Ellis Island, however, was often a long and grueling process.

81. From Samuel Ellis its last private owner. Ellis was a New York merchant who, for many years to follow, tried unsuccessfully to sell the island.

This island first was known to the American Indians by the name of Kioshk, or Gull Island, named for the birds that were its only inhabitants for years.

During the 1700s the island was known as Gibbet Island because of the criminals and pirates who were executed by being hung from gibbet trees.

When John dies in 1794, he was still the rightful owner of the island. In his will he left the island to his next born, male grandchild, under the condition that he be named after him. Since the next grandchild was in fact a girl, family members quarreled over ownership of the island. Thankfully, on April 21, 1794, the island was placed into the ownership of the city of New York.

82. President Dwight D. Eisenhower

On July 30, 1956, two years after pushing to have the phrase "under God" inserted into the pledge of allegiance, President Dwight D. Eisenhower signs a law officially declaring "In God We Trust" to be the nation's official motto.

83. E pluribus unum Latin for "Out of many, one is a traditional motto of the United States, appearing on the Great Seal.

The meaning of the phrase originates from the concept that out of the union of the original Thirteen Colonies emerged a new single nation. It is emblazoned across the scroll and clenched in the eagle's beak on the Great Seal of the United States.
The 13-letter motto was suggested in 1776 by Pierre Eugene du Simitiere to the committee responsible for developing the seal.

84. It allowed for the mass construction of tens of thousands of interstate highways in the U.S.

It was also known as the National Interstate and Defense Highways Act. It was enacted on June 29, 1956, when President Dwight D. Eisenhower signed the bill into law. With an original authorization of $25 billion for the construction of 41,000 miles (66,000 km) of the Interstate Highway System over a 10-year period, it was the largest public works project in American history through that time.

85. NASA

NASA was created in response to the Soviet Union's launch of its first satellite, Sputnik I on October 4, 1957. The 183-pound, basketball-sized satellite orbited the earth in 98 minutes.

86. Alaska and Hawaii

87. The US bought Alaska from Russia in 1867.

Edouard de Stoeckl, Russian minister to the United States, negotiated for the Russians. On March 30, 1867, the two parties agreed that the United States would pay Russia $7.2 million for the territory of Alaska.

For less than 2 cents an acre, the United States acquired nearly 600,000 square miles. This purchase ended Russia's presence in North America and ensured U.S. access to the Pacific northern rim.

88. The Kingdom of Hawai'i was sovereign from 1810 until 1893 when the monarchy was overthrown by resident American and European capitalists and landholders.

Hawai'i was an independent republic from 1894 until August 12, 1898, when it officially became a territory of the United States.

89. "In God We Trust"

By the 1950s, America was embroiled in a cold war with the Soviet Union. Fearing the spread of communism, political leaders appealed to the faith of the nation to set the U.S. apart from the godless ideology of the Soviets. Billy Graham urged President Dwight Eisenhower to direct the nation's attention toward "faith, freedom, and free enterprise."

A deeply religious man himself, Eisenhower readily complied, signing into law a bill that required "In God We Trust" to be printed on all coin and paper currency.

90. 1864

On April 22, 1864, the United States Congress passed an act allowing for "In God We Trust" to begin appearing on U.S. coins. From 1864 until 1938 it appeared on various U.S. coins, each for a different duration. It has appeared on the penny since 1909, the dime since 1916, and on all gold coins, silver dollars, half dollars, and quarter-dollar coins since 1908.

91. USA's first seven astronauts They are also referred to as the Original Seven and Astronaut Group 1.

On April 9, 1959, NASA introduces them to the press: Scott Carpenter, L. Gordon Cooper Jr., John H. Glenn Jr., Virgil "Gus" Grissom, Walter Schirra Jr., Alan Shepard Jr. and Donald Slayton. The seven men, all military test pilots, were carefully selected from a group of 32 candidates to take part in *Project Mercury,* America's first manned space program. NASA planned to begin manned orbital flights in 1961.

In January 1959, NASA began the astronaut selection procedure, screening the records of 508 military test pilots and choosing 110 candidates.

The final 31 candidates underwent various tortures that tested their tolerance of physical and psychological stress. Among other tests, the candidates were forced to spend an hour in a pressure chamber that simulated an altitude of 65,000 feet, and two hours in a chamber that was heated to 130 degrees Fahrenheit.

92. The Berlin Wall

For nearly 30 years, Berlin was divided not just by ideology, but by a concrete barrier that snaked through the city, serving as an ugly symbol of the Cold War.

Erected in haste and torn down in protest, the Berlin Wall was almost 27 miles long and was protected with barbed wire, attack dogs, and 55,000 landmines. But though the wall stood between 1961 and 1989, it could not survive a massive democratic movement that ended up bringing down the socialist German Democratic Republic (GDR) and spurring on the Cold War's end.

93. The Peace Corps

Since it was founded during the height of the Cold War, the Peace Corps was often subject to speculation that it was a front organization for the Central Intelligence Agency. The Kennedy administration ordered the CIA not to meddle in the Peace Corps' affairs, but many host countries still believed rumors and Soviet propaganda that the program's volunteers were undercover spies.

94. James Meredith

James Meredith officially became the first African American student at the University of Mississippi on October 2, 1962. He was guarded twenty-four hours a day by reserve U.S. deputy marshals and army troops, and he endured constant verbal harassment from a minority of students.

95. Shortly after noon on November 22, 1963, President John F. Kennedy was assassinated as he rode in a motorcade through Dealey Plaza in downtown Dallas, Texas by Lee Harvey Oswald.

96. The Zone Improvement Plan (ZIP)

ZIP codes are only 52 years old. The concept that was introduced during World War II when the postal service lost a huge portion of their staff who went to fight in the war. Because of this, they needed a simple way to help the understaffed postal service deliver mail effectively. It was officially implemented in 1963.

Initially, the zip code was only a two-digit number: the first denoted the city, the second denoted the state. But as the need for delivery expanded, so did the concept of the zip code. As of 1963, zip codes' numbers are determined by a few factors: the area, the regional postal facility, and the local zone.

97. They brought Tang along on their missions.

Around the same time footage started appearing in Tang commercials and NASA images appeared in print ads. The relationship continued into the Apollo program with Tang sponsoring TV coverage of Apollo 8, the first manned mission to the Moon.

98. Sears

NASA wanted that information kept secret. NASA made Tang cool. But when Apollo 11 whirled into orbit, NASA didn't want another advertising campaign based on the astronauts' use of a commercial product.

99. In 1964, President Johnson signed the Civil Rights Act.

Also, in 1965, the Voting Rights Act halted efforts to keep minorities from voting and in 1968 the Fair Housing Act of 1968 ended discrimination in renting and selling homes.

100. Mariner 4 and it took 21 grainy black and white images of Mars

Decades before Spirit and Opportunity were launched, a probe named Mariner 4 lifted off from Cape Canaveral, Fla. On July 14, 1965, it reached the planet Mars and took the first photos humans had ever seen of another world: 21 grainy black and white images, sent back through the distances of space.

101. Who did John F. Kennedy defeat in the US Presidential election in 1960?

102. The NRG Astrodome is the world's first multi-purpose, domed sports stadium. Where is it located?

103. In 1969 Congress passed the Public Health Cigarette Smoking Act (Public Law 91–222). What did it state?

104. Who was the Supreme Court's first African American justice?

105. Which South African leader was sentenced to life in prison in 1964?

106. Cult members murdered several people in August of 1969. Who was their leader?

107. In 1967, Dr. Christian Barnard performed the first transplant of what organ in South Africa?

108. Which political organization was formed in 1966 in Oakland, California as a revolutionary organization with an ideology of Black nationalism?

109. Burundi gained its independence in 1962. From what country?

110. What was the name of the first weather satellite launched by the US in 1960?

111. In what year did The People's Republic of China test its first hydrogen bomb?

112. Why did Soviet Union's astronaut Aleksei Leonov become known for in 1965?

113. Which famous American penitentiary closed in 1963? Tip: it was located in the San Francisco Bay.

114. Which Pope became the first to visit the United States in 1965?

115. Which civil rights leader was assassinated by James Earl Ray?

116. What was NASA's first manned mission?

117. What was the name of Reagan's famous 1964 speech that launched his political career as a conservative icon?

118. Why did Yuri Gagarin from the Soviet Union onboard of spacecraft Vostok 1 become famous for?

119. Which actor became the first African American and first Bahamian to win the Academy Award (Oscar) for best actor in 1964? Can you also name the movie?

120. What was the name of the unsuccessful Cuban invasion attempt that tried to overthrow Fidel Castro in 1961?

121. Which African countries gained independence from France in 1960? (There are several answers).

122. What president signed the Voting Rights Act in 1965 into a law in the US?

123. In 1963 Martin Luther King Jr. delivered a speech that would play an important role in helping pass the 1964 Civil Rights Act. What is the name given to this speech?

124. Who discovered the first quasar in 1961 in California?

125. Who assassinated Robert Kennedy in Los Angeles, California in 1968?

126. The 1966 purge of intellectuals in China by leader Mao Zedong is known as what?

127. In what year did Neil Armstrong become the first man to set foot on the moon?

128. On the same note, which was the name of this mission?

129. Which countries are the original members of the OPEC (Organization of Petroleum Exporting Countries) formed in 1960?

130. The Cuban Missile Crisis involved a stand-off between which two countries that nearly ended in nuclear war in 1962?

131. What 1964 incident triggered the official start of the Vietnam War?

132. The slogan "Flower Power" was used during the late 60s and early 70s. In opposition to which war was it created? Which poet coined the term?

133. What was Dr Martin Luther King Jr protesting in Selma Alabama?

134. In what year was Egypt's Aswan Dam completed?

135. What's the name of the 8-inch flexible magnetic disk in a square case that was introduced in 1971? Tip: It was read-only.

136. What problem did Apollo 13 face while returning to Earth?

137. What was the first jumbo jet introduced in 1970? Which airline introduced it?

138. Four Kent State University students were killed and nine were injured on May 4, 1970, during a protest. What is the name of the protest? And what was the protest about?

139. "Old Enough to Fight, Old Enough to Vote". Became a widespread slogan that eventually gave birth to the 26th Amendment. What did it accomplish and why was it passed?

140. Who released the first microprocessor in 1971?

141. Which scandal from 1972 to 1974 led to Nixon's resignation?

142. America's first space station is successfully launched into an orbit around the earth on May 14, 1974. What was it called?

143. The barcode symbology used worldwide for tracking trade items in stores *was* introduced in 1974. What is it called?

144. The Paris Peace Accords were signed in January 1973. What did they accomplish?

145. On September 17, 1976, NASA unveiled its first space shuttle to the public. What was its name?

146. On the same note. Do you know why it was called Enterprise?

147. On September 7, 1977, President Jimmy Carter and Panamanian Chief of Government Omar Torrijos signed the Panama Canal Treaty and Neutrality Treaty. What did these treaties promise?

148. The TAPS pipeline is an oil transportation system built in the US. In which state is it?

149. Physician Raymond Damadian invented a machine that could distinguish between healthy and cancerous cells and in 1977, the inventor performed the first full-body scan of a human with this machine. How do we call this device today?

150. World's first tube baby was born on July 25, 1978. What is her name?

ANSWERS 101 - 150

US & WORLD HISTORY

101. Richard Nixon

John F. Kennedy, a Democratic senator from Massachusetts, was elected president in 1960, defeating Vice President Richard Nixon. Though he clearly won the electoral vote, Kennedy's received only 118,000 more votes than Nixon in this close election.

In his inaugural address, Kennedy said, "Let the word go forth . . . that the torch has been passed to a new generation of Americans-born in this century, tempered by war, disciplined by a hard and bitter peace, proud of our ancient heritage.

102. Houston, Texas

Also known as the Houston Astrodome or simply the Astrodome. It was financed by Roy Hofheinz, mayor of Houston. Construction on the stadium began in 1962, and it officially opened in 1965.

It served as home to the Houston Astros of Major League Baseball (MLB) from its opening until 1999, and the home to the Houston Oilers of the National Football League (NFL) from 1968 until 1996, and also the part-time home of the Houston Rockets of the National Basketball Association (NBA) from 1971 until 1975.

103. This law states two things mainly:

1. It prohibited cigarette advertising on television and radio and 2. It required that each cigarette package contain the label "Warning: The Surgeon General Has Determined That Cigarette Smoking Is Dangerous to Your Health."

104. Thurgood Marshal

In 1961, Marshall was appointed by then-President John F. Kennedy to the U.S. Court of Appeals for the Second Circuit, a position he held until 1965, when Kennedy's successor, Lyndon B. Johnson, named him solicitor general.

Following the retirement of Justice Tom Clark in 1967, President Johnson appointed Marshall to the Supreme Court, a decision confirmed by the Senate with a 69-11 vote.
He would remain on the Supreme Court for 24 years before retiring for health reasons.

105. Nelson Mandela

Nelson Mandela, leader of the movement to end South African apartheid, was released from prison after 27 years on February 11, 1990.

Mandela spent the first 18 of his 27 years in jail at the brutal Robben Island Prison. Confined to a small cell without a bed or plumbing, he was forced to do hard labor in a quarry. He could write and receive a letter once every six months, and once a year he was allowed to meet with a visitor for 30 minutes.

He was later moved to another location, where he lived under house arrest.

106. Charles Manson

Charles Milles Manson was an American criminal and musician who led the Manson Family, a cult based in California, in the late 1960s. Some of the members committed a series of nine murders at four locations in July and August 1969.

107. Heart Transplant

On December 3, 1967, 53-year-old Louis Washkansky receives the first human heart transplant at Groote Schuur Hospital in Cape Town, South Africa carried out by the South African surgeon, Dr. Christian Barnard.

108. The Black Panthers

The Black Panther Party for Self-Defense (BPP) was founded in October 1966 in Oakland, California by Huey P. Newton and Bobby Seale, who met at Merritt College in Oakland. It was a revolutionary organization with an ideology of Black nationalism, socialism, and armed self-defense, particularly against police brutality.

109. Belgium

Burundi, a country located east of the Democratic Republic of Congo (DRC) gained its independence on 01 July 1962. Formerly part of German East Africa, Burundi gained its independence under the leadership of Mwami Mwambutsa IV, a Tutsi

110. TIROS-1

On the evening of April 1, 1960, President Dwight Eisenhower saw the first image sent back from space by the Television InfraRed Observation Satellite (TIROS) 1 weather satellite-shaped, as some quipped, like "an enormous hatbox." As he considered the grainy black and white image of cloud cover over the eastern United States and Canada, he remarked "the Earth doesn't look so big when you see that curvature."

111. 1967

On June 17, 1967, the People's Republic of China announced a successful hydrogen bomb test, becoming the world's fourth thermonuclear power after the US, Soviet Union and UK – but ahead of France.

112. He became the first man to go outside of a space vehicle in a "Space Walk".

On 18 March 1965, he became the first person to conduct a spacewalk, exiting the capsule during the Voskhod 2 mission for 12 minutes and 9 seconds. He was also selected to be the first Soviet person to land on the Moon although the project was cancelled.

In July 1975, Leonov commanded the Soyuz capsule in the Apollo-Soyuz mission, which docked in space for two days with an American Apollo capsule.

113. Alcatraz, The Rock

Alcatraz Prison in San Francisco's Bay closed down and transferred its last prisoners on March 21, 1963. At its peak period of use in 1950s, "The Rock," or "America's Devil Island," housed over 200 inmates at the maximum-security facility. Alcatraz remains an icon of American prisons for its harsh conditions and record for being inescapable.

Alcatraz was first explored by Juan Manuel de Ayala in 1775, who called it Isla de los Alcatraces (Pelicans) because of all the birds that lived there. It was sold in 1849 to the U.S. government. The first lighthouse in California was on Alcatraz. It became a Civil War fort and then a military prison in 1907.

114. Pope Paul VI

On this day in 1965, Pope Paul VI made a one-day visit to the United States. In doing so, he became the first pontiff to visit the Western Hemisphere

115. Martin Luther King Jr.

At 6:05 p.m. on Thursday, 4 April 1968, Martin Luther King was shot dead while standing on a balcony outside his second-floor room at the Lorraine Motel in Memphis, Tennessee. News of King's assassination prompted major outbreaks of racial violence, resulting in more than 40 deaths nationwide and extensive property damage in over 100 American cities.

116. Apollo 7

Apollo 7, the first manned Apollo mission, is launched with astronauts Walter M. Schirra, Jr.; Donn F. Eisele; and Walter Cunningham aboard. Under the command of Schirra, the crew of *Apollo 7* conducted an 11-day orbit of Earth, during which the crew transmitted the first live television broadcasts from orbit.

This mission saw the resumption of human spaceflight by the agency after the fire that killed the three Apollo 1 astronauts during a launch rehearsal test on January 27, 1967.

117. "A Time for Choosing", also known as "The Speech",

It was a speech presented during the 1964 U.S. presidential election campaign by future president Ronald Reagan on behalf of Republican candidate Barry Goldwater. Reagan was elected as governor of California in 1966.

118. He became the first man in space.

He was a Soviet pilot and cosmonaut who became the first human to journey into outer space. Travelling in the Vostok 1 capsule, Gagarin completed one orbit of Earth on 12 April 1961.

By achieving this major milestone in the Space Race, he became an international celebrity, and was awarded many medals and titles, including Hero of the Soviet Union, his nation's highest honor.

119. Sidney Poitier for "Lillies of the Field".

On April 13, 1964, Sidney Poitier becomes the first African American and first Bahamian to win the Academy Award for Best Actor, for his role as a construction worker who helps build a chapel in "Lilies of the Field" (1963).

120. The Bay of Pigs Invasion

The Bay of Pigs invasion begins when a CIA-financed and trained group of Cuban refugees lands in Cuba and attempts to topple the communist government of Fidel Castro. The attack was an utter failure. Fidel Castro had been a concern to U.S. policymakers since he seized power in Cuba with a revolution in January 1959.

121. Togo, Central African Republic, Cote D'Ivore, Senegal, Benin, Chad, and Mauritania.

Since the end of the Second World War, unlike Britain, France had devised policies to maintain its firm grip over African colonies. To that end, it had reorganized its empire in Africa to create the French Union in 1946. In 1958, the French Union was replaced with the French Community.

It was expected that eventually, these colonies would attain independence and govern their own affairs. However, despite the stated objective of autonomy within the French Community, France retained effective control over the foreign, defense and economic policies of the colonies.

After the launch of the French Community in 1958, French Guinea and Mali had opted for independence. France had accepted their demand and hoped to preserve the rest of the colonies in the Community. However, by granting independence to these two states, inadvertently, the process of dissolution of the French empire in Africa began.

122. President Lyndon B. Johnson

This act was signed into law on August 6, 1965, by President Lyndon Johnson. It outlawed the discriminatory voting practices adopted in many southern states after the Civil War, including literacy tests as a prerequisite to voting

123. "I Have a Dream" speech

On August 28, 1963, Martin Luther King Jr., delivered a speech to a massive group of civil rights marchers gathered around the Lincoln memorial in Washington DC.
King's "Dream" speech would play an important role in helping pass the 1964 Civil Rights Act, and the pivotal Selma to Montgomery march that he led in 1965 would provide momentum for the passage later that year of the Voting Rights Act.

124. Allan Sandage

Until the development of radio astronomy in the 1940s, our knowledge of the universe outside our own solar system was pretty much restricted to objects that emitted light in or near the visible spectrum. Then, astronomers began discovering objects that emitted radio waves.

In 1963, a definite identification of the radio source 3C 48 with an optical object was published by the scientists Allan Sandage and Thomas A. Matthews. Astronomers had detected what appeared to be a faint blue star at the location of the radio source and obtained its spectrum. Considerable discussion took place over what these objects might be. They were described as "quasi-stellar [meaning star-like] radio sources", or "quasi-stellar objects" (QSOs), a name which reflected their unknown nature, and this became shortened to "quasar".

125. Sirhan Sirhan

Around 12:15 a.m. PDT on June 5, 1968, Sirhan fired a 22 LR Iver-Johnson Cadet revolver at United States Senator Robert F. Kennedy and the crowd surrounding him in the Ambassador Hotel in Los Angeles, shortly after Kennedy had finished addressing supporters in the hotel's main ballroom.

126. The Cultural Revolution

During the Red August 1966, in Beijing alone 1,772 people were murdered, many of the victims were teachers who were attacked and even killed by their own students. In Shanghai, there were 704 suicides and 534 deaths related to the Cultural Revolution in September.

127. 1969

On July 20, 1969, American astronauts Neil Armstrong (1930-2012) and Edwin "Buzz" Aldrin (1930-) became the first humans ever to land on the moon.

128. Apollo 11

Fun fact: While the Apollo Guidance Computer systems that powered Neil Armstrong, Buzz Aldrin, and Michael Collins to the moon and back in July 1969 were cutting-edge for the time, they're technologically primitive compared to the cell phones and smartwatches we use half a century later.

Today's Samsung Galaxy S10 Smartphone6, with its eight gigabytes of memory, is light years ahead of the Apollo 11's computer, which propelled our fearless astronauts to the moon and back with only two kilobytes.

129. Iran, Iraq, Kuwait, Saudi Arabia, and Venezuela are all original members.

The Organization of the Petroleum Exporting Countries (OPEC) is a permanent, intergovernmental Organization, created at the Baghdad Conference on September 10–14, 1960, by Iran, Iraq, Kuwait, Saudi Arabia and Venezuela.

130. The United States and Soviet Union

The Cuban Missile Crisis of October 1962 was a direct and dangerous confrontation between the United States and the Soviet Union during the Cold War and was the moment when the two superpowers came closest to nuclear conflict.

131. The sinking of the US Destroyer Maddox by North Vietnamese Missiles in the Gulf of Tonkin

The Gulf of Tonkin Incident occurred in August 1964. North Vietnamese warships purportedly attacked United States warships, the U.S.S. Maddox and the U.S.S. C. Turner Joy, on two separate occasions in the Gulf of Tonkin, a body of water neighboring modern-day Vietnam.

132. It originated as a symbolic action of protest against the Vietnam War by poet Allen Ginsberg.

In a November 1965 essay titled "How to Make a March/Spectacle", poet Allen Ginsberg advocated that protesters should be provided with "masses of flowers" to hand out to policemen, press, politicians, and spectators.

Ginsberg wanted to counter the "specter" of the Hells Angels motorcycle gang who supported the war, equated war protesters with communists and had threatened to violently disrupt planned anti-war demonstrations at the University of California, Berkeley.

Using Ginsberg's methods, the protest received positive attention and the use of "flower power" became an integral symbol in the counterculture movement.

133. This protest was a Black voter registration campaign.

In early 1965, Martin Luther King Jr. and the SCLC decided to make Selma, located in Dallas County, Alabama, the focus of a Black voter registration campaign. King had won the Nobel Peace Prize in 1964, and his profile would help draw international attention to the events that followed.

134. 1970

After 11 years of construction, the Aswan High Dam across the Nile River in Egypt is completed on July 21, 1970. More than two miles long at its crest, the massive $1 billion dam ended the cycle of flood and drought in the Nile River region, and exploited a tremendous source of renewable energy, but had a controversial environmental impact.

135. The floppy disk

When introduced by IBM in 1971, the floppy disk enabled people to share data and programs more easily.

Computer viruses are very common now and have different sources. However, floppy disks were the first source of computer virus transmission. A malware called Elk Cloner was developed by 15-year-old Rich Skrenta in 1982.

In April 2010, Sony, the only company still producing floppy disks, announced it would stop manufacturing them in March 2011. In response to this announcement, BBC News Magazine asked readers how they use floppy disks today. Many people responded that they still use floppy disks to update or back up old systems, but others have found more unique uses as drink coasters, spatulas, ice scrapers and clothing accessories.

136. It was supposed to land in the Fra Mauro area. An explosion on board forced Apollo 13 to circle the moon without landing. The Fra Mauro site was reassigned to Apollo 14.

Apollo 13 was launched on April 11, 1970, and it was the seventh crewed mission in the Apollo space program and the third meant to land on the Moon.

The astronauts and mission control were faced with enormous logistical problems in stabilizing the spacecraft and its oxygen supply, as well as running on batteries due to the loss of the fuel cells to allow successful reentry into Earth's atmosphere.

137. A Boeing 747 which entered service with Pan Am.

It entered service with Pan Am on January 22, 1970. The 747 was the first airplane dubbed "Jumbo Jet", the first wide-body airliner.

It was a 747, originally named Clipper Victor but which Pan Am quickly re-christened Clipper Young America, which carried 335 passengers and 20 crew members from New York's JFK Airport to London Heathrow on the first commercial flight of a 747.

138. The Kent State shootings, also known as the May 4 massacre and the Kent State massacre. Students were protesting the bombing of Cambodia by United States military forces.

Students clashed with Ohio National Guardsmen on the Kent State University campus. When the Guardsmen shot and killed four students on May 4, the Kent State Shootings became the focal point of a nation deeply divided by the Vietnam War.

139. In 1971, the 26th Amendment to the United States Constitution lowered the voting age of U.S. citizens from 21 to 18 years old.

Sentiment to lower the nation's voting age dates to WWII. As American involvement in the war increased, President Roosevelt sought to increase the size of the nation's military and lowered the draft age of young men from 21 to 18 years old. Many were dismayed at the notion that if young men could fight and die for their country, they could not participate in its fundamental democratic process - voting.
On July 5th, 1971, in a ceremony in the White House East Room, in front of the 500-member choral group Young Americans in Concert, President Richard Nixon signed the certified amendment.

140. Intel Corporation

The Intel 4004 is a 4-bit central processing unit (CPU) released by Intel Corporation in 1971. Sold for US$60, it was the first commercially produced microprocessor, and the first in a long line of Intel CPUs.

141. Watergate scandal

The scandal stemmed from the Nixon administration's continual attempts to cover up its involvement in the June 17, 1972, break-in of the Democratic National Committee headquarters at the Washington, D.C., Watergate Office Building.

142. Skylab

It spent six years orbiting Earth until its decaying orbit caused it to re-enter the atmosphere. It scattered debris over the Indian Ocean and sparsely settled on areas of Western Australia.

143. The Universal Product Code (UPC or UPC code)

UPC codes are the 12-digit numbers found under barcodes on any point-of-sale product. They are made up of a company prefix, an item reference number, and a check digit.

The U.P.C. made its first commercial appearance on a package of Wrigley's Juicy Fruit chewing gum sold in Marsh's Supermarket in Troy, Ohio in June 1974.

144. The United States, South Vietnam, Viet Cong and North Vietnam formally sign "An Agreement Ending the War and Restoring Peace in Vietnam" in Paris.

The agreement's provisions were immediately and frequently broken by both North and South Vietnamese forces with no official response from the United States. Two years later, a massive North Vietnamese offensive conquered South Vietnam on April 30, 1975, after which the two countries, separated since 1954, united once more on July 2, 1976, as the Socialist Republic of Vietnam.

145. The Space Shuttle Enterprise

The unveiling took place during a public ceremony in Palmdale, California. In 1977, the Enterprise became the first space shuttle to fly on its own.

146. It was named after TV science fiction series Star Trek vehicle Enterprise.

Fans of Star Trek mounted a determined write-in campaign, before the age of the Internet and social media, to NASA and to President Gerald R. Ford to instead name this first vehicle Enterprise, after the fictional starship made famous by the show.

147. To give control of the canal to the Panamanians by the year 2000.

The United States acquired the rights to build and operate the Panama Canal during the first years of the 20th century. The Hay-Herrán Treaty, negotiated with Colombia in 1903, allowed the United States rights to the land surrounding the planned canal. The Colombian Senate refused to ratify the treaty, but Panama was in the process of seceding from Colombia.

President Theodore Roosevelt therefore supported the cause of Panamanian independence with the Canal in mind. His support paid off, and on November 18, 1903, the United States signed the Hay-Bunau-Varilla Treaty, establishing permanent U.S. rights to a Panama Canal Zone that stretched across the isthmus.

148. Alaska

The discovery of oil on Alaska's North Slope in 1968 spurred the creation of a safe and efficient way to bring those reserves to market.

Trans-Alaska Pipeline, in full **Trans-Alaska Pipeline System**, pipeline connects the oil fields of Prudhoe Bay in northern Alaska, U.S., with the harbor at Valdez, 800 miles (1,300 km) to the south.

On Nov. 16, 1973, President Nixon signed the Trans-Alaska Pipeline Authorization Act into law and on June 20, 1977, oil began to flow through the pipeline.

149. MRI or Magnetic Resonance Imaging Scanner.

The first human scan was performed by Peter Mansfield's team in Nottingham in 1976 on fellow author Andrew Maudsley's finger. However, on July 3, 1977, the first MRI body exam was performed on a human being by Damadian and his team.

150. Louise Joy Brown

She is an English woman who was the first human to have been born after conception by in vitro fertilization experiment (IVF).

She was born at Oldham General Hospital, Lancashire, by planned Caesarean section. Her parents, Lesley and John Brown, had been trying to conceive naturally for nine years, but Lesley faced complications of blocked fallopian tubes. Although the media referred to Brown as a "test tube baby", her conception actually took place in a Petri dish.

Her younger sister, Natalie Brown, was also conceived through IVF four years later, and became the world's 40th child after conception by IVF. In May 1999, Natalie was the first human born after conception by IVF to give birth herself without IVF.

151. What happened at Three Mile Island in Pennsylvania in1979?

152. In 1979, President Jimmy Carter allowed Iran's deposed Shah, a pro-Western autocrat who had been expelled from his country some months before to come to the United States for cancer treatment. This action triggered a hostage situation directly affecting US citizens. What was this crisis called? What was it about?

153. Who became the first woman to be UK Prime Minister in 1979?

154. On the same note, who was the first female Prime Minister in the world?

155. The Second Indochina War is one of the many nicknames given to this war. It has been the only conflict that ended in defeat for the USA. Which war is it?

156. Which Nobel Prize did Amnesty International win in 1977?

157. On March 27, 1980, a natural disaster affected Skamania County, *Washington*, United *States*. What type of disaster was it?

158. In 1980, the US led a boycott to protest the 1979 Soviet invasion of Afghanistan. What did the US and other 65 countries boycott?

159. What new autoimmune disease was discovered in 1981?

160. Who was the first woman nominated to the Supreme Court? Which president nominated her?

161. On June 18, 1983, the space shuttle *Challenger* is launched into space on its second mission. On board the shuttle was the first American woman to travel into space. Who was it?

162. The first word-processor software was launched in 1983 by which company?

163. On 31 October 1984, India's Prime Minister was killed by her Sikh bodyguards. Who was she?

164. The first version of Microsoft Windows was released in 1985. What was the name of this version?

165. On 26 April 1986 a nuclear accident occurred in reactor 4 of a plant located in the north of Ukrainian SSR in the Soviet Union. How is this disaster called?

166. On January 28, 1986, the US space program suffered a fatal incident with one of their Space Shuttles. What was this fatal incident?

167. On the same note, who was Christa McAuliffe and how is she related to this terrible accident?

168. When and where was Mad Cow Disease (BSE - Bovine Spongiform Encephalopathy) first diagnosed?

169. He would have been the first Greek American President but lost the 1988 election to his Republican opponent George H. W. Bush, who was the sitting Vice President at the time. What is his name?

170. This was a protracted armed conflict between Iran and Iraq that began on 22 September 1980 with the Iraqi invasion of Iran by Saddam Hussein. It lasted for almost eight years and ended on 20 August 1988, following the acceptance of United Nations Security Council Resolution 598 by both sides. This conflict is known as..?

151. Unit 2 reactor at The Three Mile Island nuclear plant partially melted down on March 28, 1979.

This error resulted in the release of a small amount of radioactive material. Experts determined that the approximately 2 million people in the nearby area during the accident were exposed to small amounts of radiation.

Three Mile Island's Unit 1 continued operation for 40 years before shutting down in the fall of 2019.

152. The Iran Hostage Crisis

On November 4, 1979, a group of Iranian students stormed the U.S. Embassy in Tehran, taking more than 60 American hostages.

The source of tension between Iran and the U.S. stemmed from an increasingly intense conflict over oil. British and American corporations had controlled Iran's petroleum reserves almost since their discovery. In 1951 Iran's newly elected prime minister announced a plan to nationalize the country's oil industry. The American C.I.A. and the British intelligence secretly overthrew Mossadegh and replace him with a member of Iran's royal family named Mohammed Reza Shah Pahlavi.

The Shah turned out to be a brutal arbitrary dictator and many Iranians were fed up with his government. In protest, they turned to Ayatollah Ruhollah Khomeini, a radical cleric.

In July 1979, the revolutionaries forced the Shah to disband his government and flee to Egypt. The Ayatollah installed a militant Islamist government in its place.

In October 1979 President Carter agreed to allow the exiled leader to enter the U.S. for treatment of an advanced malignant lymphoma. Anti-American sentiment in Iran exploded and this hostage crisis was one of the consequences.

153. Margaret Thatcher

She was leader of the Conservative Party, becomes Britain's first female prime minister on May 4, 1979. The Oxford-educated chemist and lawyer took office the day after the Conservatives won a 44-seat majority in general parliamentary elections.

154. The first female Prime Minister in the world was Sirimavo Bandaranaike. In 1960, she became Prime Minister of Sri Lanka (then the Dominion of Ceylon).

Sirimavo Ratwatte Dias Bandaranaike (17 April 1916 – 10 October 2000) was a Sri Lankan politician. She served as prime minister three times and was the leader of the Sri Lanka Freedom Party. She was the first female to be elected head of government in the world.

155. The Vietnam War

It has been variously called the Second Indochina War, the Vietnam Conflict, and Nam. In Vietnam it is commonly known as Kháng chiến chống Mỹ (Resistance War against America).

It was the first war to come into American living rooms nightly, and the only conflict that ended in defeat for American arms. The war caused turmoil on the home front, as anti-war protests became a feature of American life.

156. Nobel Peace Prize

Amnesty International, the worldwide organization that fights man's inhumanity to man, Monday won the 1977 Nobel Peace Prize, and the delayed 1976 prize was given to Betty Williams and Mairead Corrigan, leaders of the Northern Ireland Peace Movement.

In its citation, the Norwegian Nobel Committee said, "Amnesty International has given practical humanitarian and impartial support to people who have been imprisoned because of their race, religion or political views."

157. A series of volcanic explosions and pyroclastic flows began at *Mount St. Helens*.

Many tens of thousands of acres of prime forest, as well as recreational sites, bridges, roads, and trails, were destroyed or heavily damaged. More than 185 miles of highways and roads and 15 miles of railways were destroyed or extensively damaged. During the eruption, 57 people were killed.

158. The Summer Olympic Games in Moscow

The Olympic boycott was supported by President Carter, the US Congress and the American people but was unsuccessful at preventing the Games from being held in Moscow.

Many countries ultimately joined the US in a full boycott of the Games. These included Japan and West Germany, where Chancellor Schmidt was able to convince the West German Olympic Committee to support the boycott. China, the Philippines, Chile, Argentina and Norway also boycotted the Games entirely.

159. AIDS (Acquired Immunodeficiency Syndrome) was first identified in the United States in 1981.

In 1984, 3 years after scientists identified AIDS, they discovered its cause: HIV.
HIV (Human Immunodeficiency Virus) is a virus that attacks the body's immune system. If HIV is not treated, it can lead to AIDS (acquired immunodeficiency syndrome).

160. Sandra Day O'Connor was nominated to the Supreme Court by President Reagan.

He nominated her on August 19, 1981, thus fulfilling his 1980 campaign promise to appoint the first woman to the highest court in the United States.

161. Dr. Sally K. Ride a mission specialist

The United States had screened a group of female pilots in 1959 and 1960 for possible astronaut training but later decided to restrict astronaut qualification to men. In 1978, NASA changed its policy and announced that it had approved six women out of some 3,000 original applicants to become the first female astronauts in the U.S. space program. She was one of six women selected to enter the astronaut corps in 1978.

162. The Microsoft Corporation

Word was originally the "Bravo" product. When the first version was released in 1983, it was the first word-processing product to feature the "WYSIWYG" design philosophy that what appears on screen should appear in print. It was the first program to feature line breaks, bold-faced and italic fonts on screen, and typeset-quality printing.

163 Indira Gandhi

The assassination sparked four days of riots that left more than 8,000 Indian Sikhs dead in revenge attacks.

She was elected as prime minister of India in 1966 and, to date, the only female prime minister. Gandhi was the daughter of Jawaharlal Nehru, the first prime minister of India. She served as prime minister from January 1966 to March 1977 and again from January 1980 until her assassination in October 1984, making her the second longest-serving Indian prime minister after her father.

164. Windows 1

This is where it all started for Windows. The original Windows 1 was released in November 1985 and was Microsoft's first true attempt at a graphical user interface in 16-bit. Development was spearheaded by Microsoft founder Bill Gates and ran on top of MS-DOS, which relied on command-line input.

165. The Chernobyl disaster

As surplus energy surged through the reactor, its core combusted, immediately killing nearby workers and exposing others to deadly levels of radiation. In the nearby town of Prypiat, Ukraine, people woke up to respiratory distress and nausea. Emergency response workers encased the reactor in a concrete sarcophagus and, unprepared for exposure to radioactivity, became stricken with severe symptoms of radiation poisoning.

Tens of thousands of Soviet citizens filed into Chernobyl to help, considering it their patriotic duty; all were exposed to dangerous levels of radiation with no warning from the government. It took two days for the explosion to be announced, in vague terms, on the national news; not until Sweden discovered a radiation cloud that had drifted across Europe was the true extent of the Chernobyl explosion revealed.

166. The Space Shuttle Challenger exploded and broke apart 73 seconds into its flight, killing all seven crew members aboard.

167. High school teacher Christa McAuliffe was the first American civilian selected to go into space. She died in the explosion of the space shuttle 'Challenger' in 1986.

Christa McAuliffe, a 37-year-old high school social studies teacher from New Hampshire, won a competition that earned her a place among the seven-member crew of the *Challenger*. She underwent months of shuttle training but then, beginning January 23, was forced to wait six long days as the *Challenger*'s launch countdown was repeatedly delayed because of weather and technical problems. Finally, on January 28, the shuttle lifted off.

168. It was first diagnosed in the United Kingdom in 1985 as an outbreak of illness in cattle with death preceded by neurological signs of incoordination, weight loss, and demonstration of unusual aggression in some cases.

169. Michael Dukakis

Dukakis won 10 states and the District of Columbia, receiving a total of 111 electoral votes compared to Bush's. He received 45% of the popular vote to Bush's 53%. Many commentators blamed Dukakis' loss on the embarrassing photograph of him in a tank taken on September 13, 1988, which subsequently formed the basis of a successful Republican attack ad.

170. The Iran-Iraq War or the First Gulf War

Saddam's primary rationale for the attack against Iran cited the need to prevent Ruhollah Khomeini, who had spearheaded Iran's Islamic Revolution in 1979, from exporting the new Iranian ideology to Iraq.

STATE BIRDS, LANDMARKS, CAPITALS, FLAGS & MORE

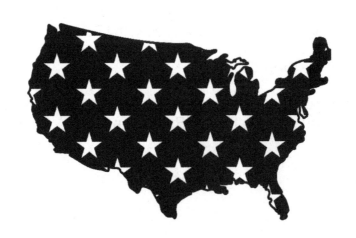

QUESTIONS 1 – 50

STATE BIRDS, LANDMARKS, CAPITALS, FLAGS & MORE

1. What is the state bird of New York?

- EASTERN BLUEBIRD
- WILD TURKEY
- NORTHERN CARDINAL
- EASTERN GOLDFINCH

2. What is the capital of Alabama?

3. In what state is the Grand Canyon located?

4. Which one of these is a state bird of Mississippi?

- SOUTHERN CARDINAL
- BOBWHITE QUAIL
- NORTHERN MOCKINGBIRD
- RED CHICKEN

5. What is the capital of Alaska?

6. In what state is the Edmund Pettus Bridge located?

7. What is the state bird of Pennsylvania?

- COMMON LOON
- LARK BUNTING
- RUFFED GROUSE
- BALD EAGLE

8. What is the capital of Arizona?

9. In what state is the Diamond Head located?

10. What is the state bird of Washington?

- LARK BUNTING
- WILLOW GOLDFINCH
- WILLOW PTARMIGAN
- CALIFORNIA VALLEY QUAIL

11. What is the capital of California?

12. In what state is the Bourbon Street located?

13. What is the state bird of Illinois?

- AMERICAN ROBIN

- PIGEON

- NORTHERN CARDINAL

- WESTERN MEADOWLARK

14. What is the capital of Connecticut?

15. In what state is the Pikes Peak located?

16. What is the state bird of New Jersey?

- PURPLE FINCH

- AMERICAN ROBIN

- EASTERN GOLDFINCH

- RUFFED GROUSE

17. What is the capital of Delaware?

18. In what state is the Portland Head Lighthouse located?

19. What is the state bird of Indiana?

- MOUNTAIN BLUEBIRD

- NORTHERN CARDINAL

- WILD TURKEY

- RUFFED GROUSE

20. What is the capital of Idaho?

21. In what state is the Fort McHenry National Monument located?

22. What is the state bird of Delaware?

- EASTERN GOLDFINCH

- BLUE HEN CHICKEN

- EASTERN BLUEBIRD

- AMERICAN ROBIN

23. What is the capital of Illinois?

24. In what state is the Monument Rocks National Natural Landmark located?

25. What is the state bird of Colorado?

- LARK BUNTING

- BLUE HEN

- AMERICAN ROBIN

26. What is the capital of Iowa?

27. In what state is the Hot Springs National Park located?

28. Which one of these is a state bird of Oklahoma?

- FALCON

- WESTERN MEADOWLARK

- EASTERN BLUEBIRD

- SCISSOR-TAILED FLYCATCHER

29. What is the capital of Kansas?

30. In what state is the Faneuil Hall located?

31. What is the state bird of Georgia?

- EASTERN BLUEBIRD

- EASTERN BROWN PELICAN

- AMERICAN ROBIN

- BROWN THRASHER

32. What is the capital of Kentucky?

33. In what state is the Mark Twain House located?

34. What is the state bird of Arkansas?

- COMMON LOON

- BROWN THRASHER

- LARK BUNTING

- NORTHERN MOCKINGBIRD

35. In what state is Silver City located?

36. Which one of these is a state bird of Massachusetts?

- NORTHERN MOCKINGBIRD

- NENE

- BLACK-CAPPED CHICKADEE

- BALD EAGLE

37. What is the capital of Maine?

38. In what city is the Mall of America located?

39. What is the state bird of West Virginia?

- RHODE ISLAND RED

- NORTHERN CARDINAL

- EASTERN BLUEBIRD

- CALIFORNIA WREN

40. In what state is the Vicksburg National Military Park located?

41. What is the state bird of Alaska?

- WILLOW PTARMIGAN

- NORTHERN MOCKINGBIRD

- CALIFORNIA VALLEY QUAIL

- BLUE HEN CHICKEN

42. What is the capital of Maryland?

43. In what state is the Mason Dixon Marker?

44. What is the state bird of Oregon?

- AMERICAN ROBIN

- EASTERN BLUEBIRD

- WESTERN MEADOWLARK

- NORTHERN CARDINAL

45. What is the capital of Michigan?

46. In what state is the Madam C.J. Walker Manufacturing Company located?

47. What is the state bird of Wisconsin?

- AMERICAN ROBIN

- NORTHERN CARDINAL

- COMMON LOON

- WOOD THRUSH

48. What is the capital of Mississippi?

49. In what state is the Hoover Dam located?

50. What is the state bird of Maryland?

- WILLOW PTARMIGAN

- WOOD THRUSH

- BLUE HEN CHICKEN

- BALTIMORE ORIOLE

ANSWERS 1 – 50
STATE BIRDS, LANDMARKS, CAPITALS, FLAGS & MORE

1. The state bird of New York is the eastern bluebird. Male eastern bluebirds have brick-red breasts. Their distinguishing characteristic is their deep blue head, feathers, and back. The female is grayer in these areas but tinged with blue.

2. Montgomery

3. Arizona

4. A state bird of Mississippi is the northern mockingbird. It has been known to imitate the songs of 20 or more species within 10 minutes. (The wood duck is Mississippi's designated waterfowl.)

5. Juneau

6. Alabama

7. The state bird of Pennsylvania is the ruffed grouse, which is sometimes called a partridge. The male is famous for drumming, beating his wings rapidly against the air, to proclaim his territory.

8. Phoenix

9. Hawaii

10. The state bird of Washington state is the willow goldfinch, also known as the American goldfinch or the eastern goldfinch. The 13-cm (5-inch) willow goldfinch is found across North America. The male is bright yellow, with black cap, wings, and tail.

11. Sacramento

12. Louisiana

13. The state bird of Illinois is the northern cardinal. The northern cardinal is the only red North American bird with a crest. It is the official bird of seven eastern U.S. states and is especially common in the southeast.

14. Hartford

15. Colorado

16. The state bird of New Jersey is the eastern goldfinch, also known as the American goldfinch. The 13-cm (5-inch) eastern goldfinch is found across North America. The male is bright yellow, with black cap, wings, and tail.

17. Dover

18. Maine

19. The state bird of Indiana is the northern cardinal. The northern cardinal is the only red North American bird with a crest. It is the official bird of seven eastern U.S. states and is especially common in the southeast.

20. Boise

21. Maryland

22. The state bird of Delaware is the blue hen chicken, or Delaware blue hen. It is one of three state birds (South Dakota and Rhode Island having the others) that is not native to the United States. It is descended primarily from the wild red jungle fowl (*Gallus gallus*) of India.

23. Springfield

24. Kansas

25. The state bird of Colorado is the lark bunting. Breeding males are black with white patches on their wings. Females and nonbreeding males are brownish.

26. Des Moines

27. Arkansas

28. One state bird of Oklahoma is the scissor-tailed flycatcher. This bird has a black-and-white deeply forked long tail. The bird is generally gray with black wings. (Oklahoma's game bird is the wild turkey.)

29. Topeka

30. Massachusetts

31. The state bird of Georgia is the brown thrasher. It is from the bird family Mimidae and is known for its singing and mimicking. The brown thrasher is a good singer but does not mimic as often as the mockingbird.

32. Frankfort

33. Connecticut

34. The state bird o Arkansas is the northern mockingbird. It has been known to imitate the songs of 20 or more species within 10 minutes.

35. Idaho

36. A state bird of Massachusetts is the black-capped chickadee. When it comes to mating, black-capped chickadees have a dominance hierarchy structure. More dominant males tend to mate with more dominant females. (The wild turkey is the state game bird.)

37. Augusta

38. Minnesota

39. The state bird of West Virginia is the northern cardinal. The northern cardinal is the only red North American bird with a crest. It is the official bird of seven eastern U.S. states and is especially common in the southeast.

40. Mississippi

41. The state bird of Alaska is the willow ptarmigan. Ptarmigan are a species of partridgelike grouse of cold regions, belonging to the genus *Lagopus* of the grouse family, Tetraonidae.

42. Annapolis

43. Delaware

44. The state bird of Oregon is the western meadowlark. Western meadowlarks have a bright yellow breast with a black V crossing it. In flight, the outer tail feathers flash white.

45. Lansing

46. Indiana

47. The state bird of Wisconsin is the American robin. The American robin is about 25 cm (10 inches) long and has gray-brown upperparts, a rusty breast, and white-tipped outer tail feathers.

48. Jackson

49. Nevada

50. The state bird of Maryland is the Baltimore oriole. The Baltimore Orioles baseball team is named after this black, white, and golden orange bird.

51. What is the capital of Missouri?

52. In what state is the Wrigley Field located?

53. What is the state bird of Vermont?

- EASTERN GOLDFINCH
- EASTERN BLUEBIRD
- AMERICAN ROBIN
- HERMIT THRUSH

54. What is the capital of Montana?

55. In what state is the Castillo de San Marcos located?

56. What is the state bird of South Dakota?

- PARROT
- HERMIT THRUSH
- RING-NECKED PHEASANT
- BLUE HEN CHICKEN

57. What is the capital of Nebraska?

58. In what state is the Rock n' Roll Hall of Fame located?

59. What is the state bird of Missouri?

- HERMIT THRUSH
- AMERICAN ROBIN
- EASTERN BLUEBIRD
- NORTHERN CARDINAL

60. What is the capital of Nevada?

61. In what state is The Flying Horse Carousel located?

62. Which one of these is a state bird of Tennessee?

- ROADRUNNER
- NORTHERN MOCKINGBIRD
- WILD TURKEY
- AMERICAN ROBIN

63. What is the capital of Ohio?

64. In what state is the Glacier National Park located?

65. What is the state bird of North Carolina?

- NENE

- YELLOWHAMMER

- BALD EAGLE

- NORTHERN CARDINAL

66. What is the capital of New Hampshire?

67. In what state is Graceland located?

68. What is the state bird of Kentucky?

- AMERICAN ROBIN

- CENTRAL CARDINAL

- NORTHERN CARDINAL

- RED CHICKEN

69. What is the capital of North Dakota?

70. In what state is the Space Needle located?

71. What is the state bird of Virginia?

- NORTHERN CARDINAL

- AMERICAN ROBIN

- PURPLE FINCH

- MOUNTAIN BLUEBIRD

72. What is the capital of Oregon?

73. In what state is the Rudyard Kipling House-Naulakha located?

74. What is the state bird of Arizona?

- COUES'S CACTUS WREN

- ROADRUNNER

- AMERICAN ROBIN

- NENE

75. What is the capital of Pennsylvania?

76. In what state is The Alamo located?

77. What is the state bird of Iowa?

- COMMON LOON
- EASTERN BLUEBIRD
- AMERICAN ROBIN
- EASTERN GOLDFINCH

78. What is the capital of South Dakota?

79. In what state is Fort Sumter located?

80. What is the state bird of Minnesota?

- ROADRUNNER
- PURPLE FINCH
- WOOD DUCK
- COMMON LOON

81. What is the capital of Vermont?

82. In what state is Washington's Crossing located?

83. What is the state bird of North Dakota?

- BROWN THRASHER
- WESTERN MEADOWLARK
- BALTIMORE ORIOLE
- GOOSE

84. What is the capital of Washington?

85. In what state is Mount Rushmore located?

86. What is the state bird of Rhode Island?

- WILLOW GOLDFINCH
- HERMIT THRUSH
- RHODE ISLAND RED
- PIGEON

87. What is the capital of West Virginia?

88. In what state is Mount Washington located?

89. Which one of these is a state bird of Alabama?

- YELLOWHAMMER
- AMERICAN ROBIN
- LARK BUNTING
- COUES'S CACTUS WREN

90. What is the capital of Wyoming?

91. In what state is the Gateway Arch located?

92. What is the state bird of New Hampshire?

- PURPLE FINCH
- RUFFED GROUSE
- SCISSOR-TAILED FLYCATCHER
- WILD TURKEY

93. What is the capital of Wisconsin?

94. In what state is the Old Faithful located?

95. What is the state bird of Louisiana?

- WOOD DUCK
- WESTERN MEADOWLARK
- WILD TURKEY
- EASTERN BROWN PELICAN

96. What is the capital of Virginia?

97. In what state is the Ebenezer Baptist Church located?

98. What is the state bird of New Mexico?

- ROADRUNNER
- WESTERN MEADOWLARK
- HERMIT THRUSH
- NORTHERN CARDINAL

99. What is the capital of South Carolina?

100. In what state is the Denali (formerly Mount McKinley) located?

101. What is the state bird of Florida?

- WESTERN MEADOWLARK
- SOUTHERN MOCKINGBIRD
- LARK BUNTING
- NORTHERN MOCKINGBIRD

102. What is the capital of North Carolina?

103. In what state is Churchill Downs located?

104. Which one of these is a state bird of South Carolina?

- EASTERN GOLDFINCH
- CAROLINA WREN
- MOUNTAIN BLUEBIRD
- WESTERN MEADOWLARK

105. What is the capital of Rhode Island?

106. In what state is the Palace of the Governors located?

107. What is the state bird of Texas?

- NORTHERN MOCKINGBIRD
- AMERICAN ROBIN
- BALD EAGLE
- HERMIT THRUSH

108. What is the capital of New York?

109. In what state is Kitty Hawk located?

110. What is the state bird of California?

- MOUNTAIN BLUEBIRD
- BLACK-CAPPED CHICKADEE
- CALIFORNIA VALLEY QUAIL
- NORTHERN CARDINAL

111. What is the capital of New Mexico?

112. In what state is Times Square located?

113. What is the state bird of Hawaii?

- PURPLE FINCH

- MOCKINGBIRD

- ROADRUNNER

- NENE

114. What is the capital of New Jersey?

115. In what state is the Price Tower located?

51. Jefferson City

52. Illinois

53. The state bird of Vermont is the hermit thrush. The hermit thrush is 18 cm (7 inches) long. It is a famous singer found in Canadian and U.S. coniferous woodlands.

54. Helena

55. Florida

56. The state bird of South Dakota is the ring-necked pheasant, also called the common pheasant. It has 20–30 races ranging across Asia. Birds naturalized elsewhere are mixtures of races in which the gray-rumped ringneck (or Chinese) strain usually dominates.

57. Lincoln

58. Ohio

59. The state bird of Missouri is the eastern bluebird. Male eastern bluebirds have brick-red breasts. Their distinguishing characteristic is their deep blue head, feathers, and back. The female is grayer in these areas but tinged with blue.

60. Carson City

61. Rhode Island

62. A state bird of Tennessee is the northern mockingbird. It has been known to imitate the songs of 20 or more species within 10 minutes. (The bobwhite quail is Tennessee's game bird.)

63. Columbus

64. Montana

65. The state bird of North Carolina is the northern cardinal. The northern cardinal is the only red North American bird with a crest. It is the official bird of seven eastern U.S. states and is especially common in the southeast.

66. Concord

67. Tennessee

68. The state bird of Kentucky is the northern cardinal. The northern cardinal is the only red North American bird with a crest. It is the official bird of seven eastern U.S. states and is especially common in the southeast.

69. Bismarck

70. Washington

71. The state bird of Virginia is the northern cardinal. The northern cardinal is the only red North American bird with a crest. It is the official bird of seven eastern U.S. states and is especially common in the southeast.

72. Salem

73. Vermont

74. The state bird of Arizona is Coues's cactus wren. The songbird's crown and hind neck are deep brown. The back is grayish brown variegated with white. The underparts are white to cinnamon-buff and are spotted black. Above each eye there is a white line.

75. Harrisburg

76. Texas

77. The state bird of Iowa is the eastern goldfinch, also known as the American goldfinch. The 13-cm (5-inch) eastern goldfinch is found across North America. The male is bright yellow, with black cap, wings, and tail.

78. Pierre

79. South Carolina

80. The state bird of Minnesota is the common loon. The common loon is known for its haunting voice, which is heard in the summer on northern lakes and is considered to be a symbol of the wilderness.

81. Montpelier

82. New Jersey

83. The state bird of North Dakota is the western meadowlark. Western meadowlarks have a bright yellow breast with a black V crossing it. In flight, the outer tail feathers flash white.

84. Olympia

85. South Dakota

86. The state bird of Rhode Island is the Rhode Island Red. The Rhode Island Red is a chicken bred for its egg laying.

87. Charleston

88. New Hampshire

89. One state bird of Alabama is locally called the yellowhammer (elsewhere called a northern, or yellow-shafted, flicker). It is a 16-cm- (6-inch-) long bird that derives its name from the yellow on its underparts, wings, tail, and head. The wild turkey is Alabama's game bird.

90. Cheyenne

91. Missouri

92. The state bird of New Hampshire is the purple finch. The male purple finch is a red pink color on the head. The belly of the purple finch is white mixed with red-pink, and the back is brown mixed with red pink. Female purple finches have no red.

93. Madison

94. Wyoming

95. The state bird of Louisiana is the eastern brown pelican. The eastern brown pelican is an endangered species with a 46-cm- (18-inch-) long bill. The feathers on its body are silver-gray. Its head is white in front and brown in back.

96. Richmond

97. Georgia

98. The state bird of New Mexico is the roadrunner. Clumsy in flight and tiring rapidly, the bird usually prefers to run along roads or across sagebrush, chaparral, or mesquite flats. Beep! Beep!

99. Columbia

100. Alaska

101. The state bird of Florida is the northern mockingbird. It has been known to imitate the songs of 20 or more species within 10 minutes.

102. Raleigh

103. Kentucky

104. One state bird of South Carolina is the Carolina wren. The Carolina wren is a small round bird with a downward-curving bill. These wrens are very protective of their territory: they chase away potential threats with their singing. (South Carolina also has a designated game bird, the wild turkey, and a designated waterfowl, the wood duck.)

105. Providence

106. New Mexico

107. The state bird of Texas is the northern mockingbird. It has been known to imitate the songs of 20 or more species within 10 minutes.

108. Albany

109. North Carolina

110. The state bird of California is the California valley quail. It is short-necked plump bird with a feather protruding from the forehead. The wings are short and broad.

111. Santa Fe

112. New York

113. The state bird of Hawaii is the nene, or Hawaiian goose. The nene is a relative of the Canada goose that evolved in the Hawaiian Islands into a nonmigratory nonaquatic species with shortened wings and half-webbed feet for walking on rough lava.

114. Trenton

115. Oklahoma

QUESTIONS
STATE BIRDS, LANDMARKS, CAPITALS, FLAGS & MORE

STATE FLAGS. Name the state.

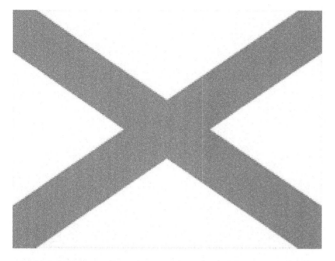

1.
- ■ CONNECTICUT
- ■ ALABAMA
- ■ MONTANA
- ■ NORTH DAKOTA

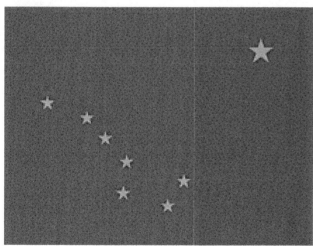

2.
- ■ NEVADA
- ■ INDIANA
- ■ ALASKA
- ■ MAINE

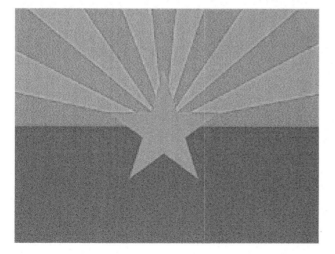

3.
- ■ ARKANSAS
- ■ ARIZONA
- ■ COLORADO
- ■ NEW MEXICO

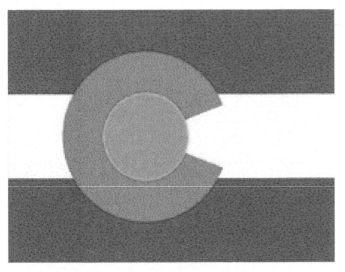

4.
- NORTH CAROLINA
- HAWAII
- COLORADO
- MISSISSIPPI

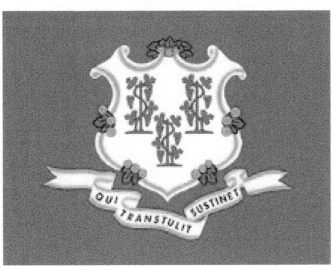

5.
- NEVADA
- MONTANA
- IDAHO
- CONNECTICUT

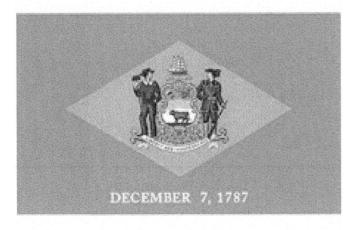

6.
- MINNESOTA
- ALASKA
- LOUISIANA
- DELAWARE

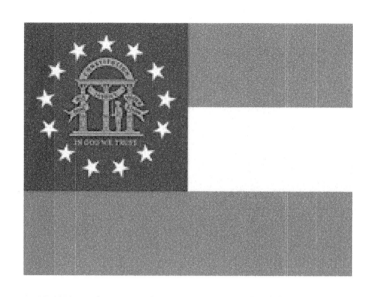

7.
- NORTH CAROLINA
- GEORGIA
- IOWA
- CALIFORNIA

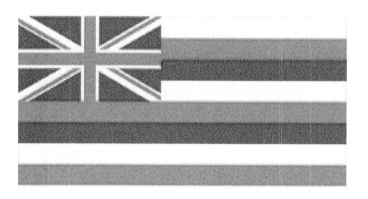

8.
- ARKANSAS
- MISSOURI
- ALABAMA
- HAWAII

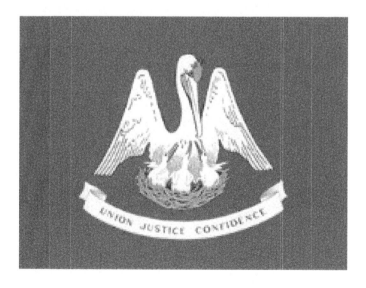

9.
- DELAWARE
- MICHIGAN
- KANSAS
- LOUISIANA

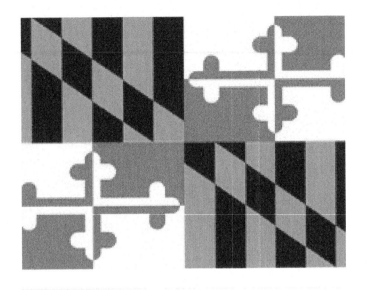

10.
- ARIZONA
- KENTUCKY
- MASSACHUSETTS
- MARYLAND

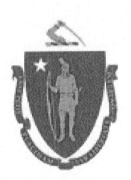

11.
- ILLINOIS
- CALIFORNIA
- MASSACHUSETTS
- FLORIDA

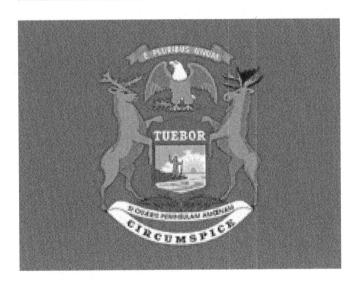

12.
- MICHIGAN
- KANSAS
- NEW YORK
- CONNECTICUT

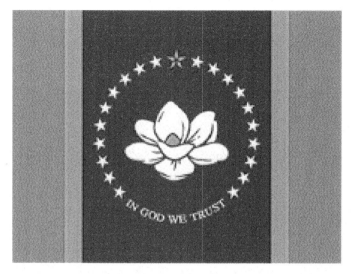

13.
- ARIZONA
- IOWA
- MISSISSIPPI
- MARYLAND

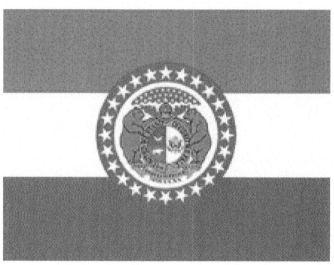

14.
- IOWA
- MISSOURI
- ARKANSAS
- NORTH CAROLINA

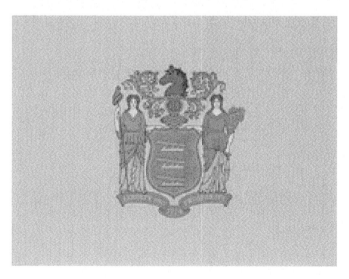

15.
- NEW MEXICO
- ARIZONA
- NEW JERSEY
- ILLINOIS

16.

- New Mexico

- California

- Massachusetts

- New Jersey

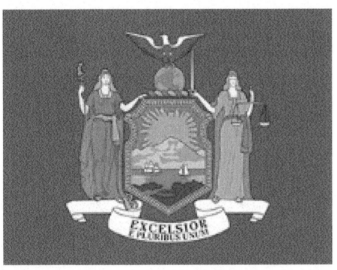

17.

- Montana

- Kansas

- Connecticut

- New York

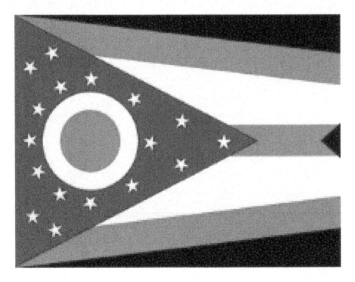

18.

- Georgia

- Ohio

- Colorado

- Mississippi

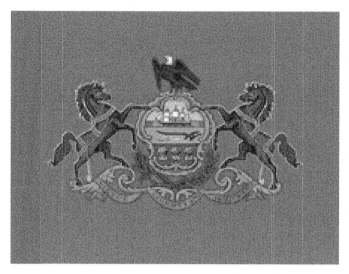

19.
- NEBRASKA
- NEW HAMPSHIRE
- NORTH DAKOTA
- PENNSYLVANIA

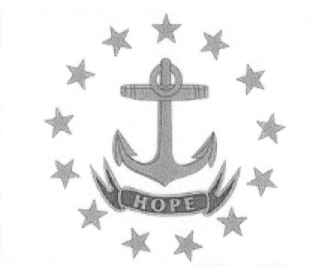

20.
- RHODE ISLAND
- ILLINOIS
- CALIFORNIA
- MASSACHUSETTS

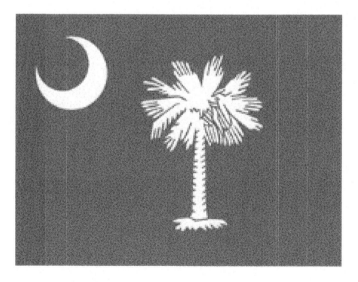

21.
- IDAHO
- LOUISIANA
- ALASKA
- SOUTH CAROLINA

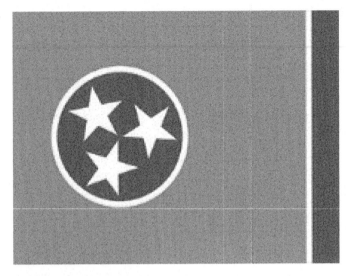

22.
- Hawaii
- North Carolina
- Iowa
- Tennessee

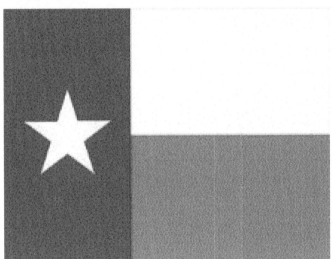

23.
- North Carolina
- Iowa
- Texas
- Georgia

ANSWERS

STATE BIRDS, LANDMARKS, CAPITALS, FLAGS & MORE

STATE FLAGS. Name the state.

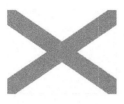

1. ALABAMA

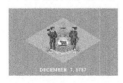

2. ALASKA

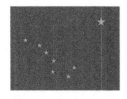

3. ARIZONA

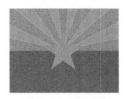

4. COLORADO

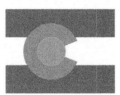

5. CONNECTICUT

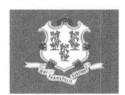

6. DELAWARE

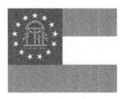

7. GEORGIA

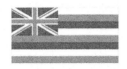

8. HAWAII

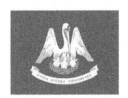

9. LOUISIANA

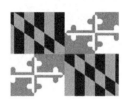

10. MARYLAND

11. MASSACHUSETTS

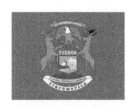

12. MICHIGAN

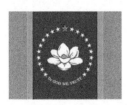

13. MISSISSIPPI

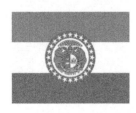

14. MISSOURI

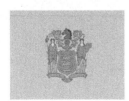

15. NEW JERSEY

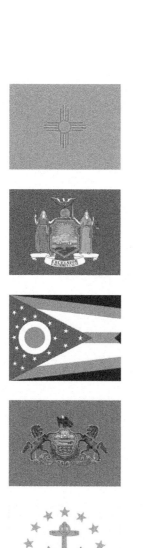

16. NEW MEXICO

17. NEW YORK

18. OHIO

19. PENNSYLVANIA

20. RHODE ISLAND

21. SOUTH CAROLINA

22. TENNESSEE

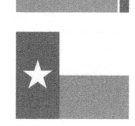

23. TEXAS

QUESTIONS

STATE BIRDS, LANDMARKS, CAPITALS, FLAGS & MORE

DO YOU RECOGNIZE THE STATE? Name the state.

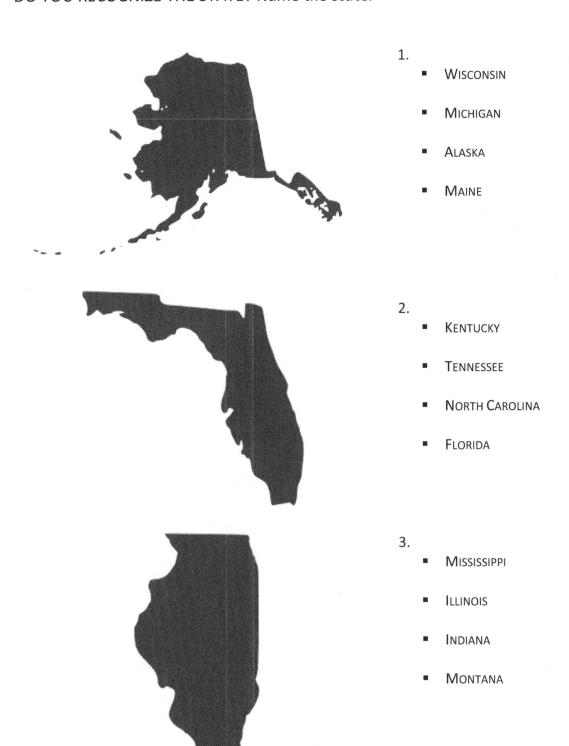

1.
- WISCONSIN
- MICHIGAN
- ALASKA
- MAINE

2.
- KENTUCKY
- TENNESSEE
- NORTH CAROLINA
- FLORIDA

3.
- MISSISSIPPI
- ILLINOIS
- INDIANA
- MONTANA

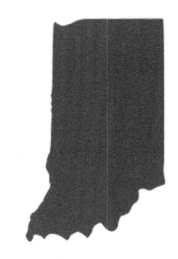

4.
- NEVADA
- WASHINGTON
- ALABAMA
- INDIANA

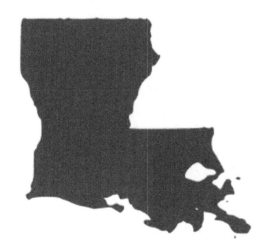

5.
- VIRGINIA
- MINNESOTA
- LOUISIANA
- OHIO

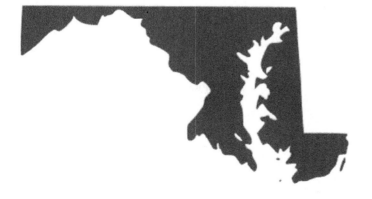

6.
- KENTUCKY
- WEST VIRGINIA
- VERMONT
- MARYLAND

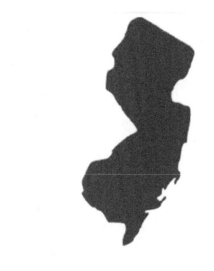

7.

- New Hampshire

- New Jersey

- Rhode Island

- Vermont

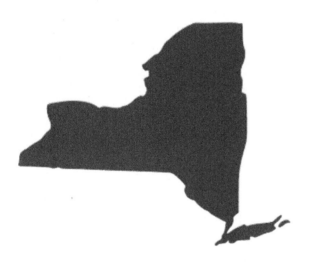

8.

- Virginia

- Louisiana

- Massachusetts

- New York

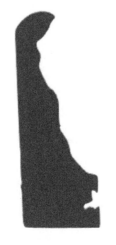

9.

- New Hampshire

- Vermont

- Delaware

- Idaho

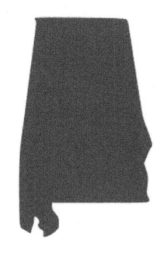

10.
- Georgia
- Iowa
- Oregon
- Alabama

11.
- Nevada
- Arkansas
- New Mexico
- Ohio

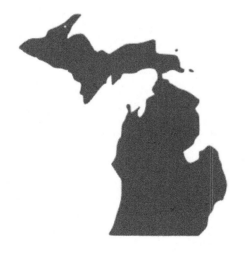

12.
- Louisiana
- Maryland
- West Virginia
- Michigan

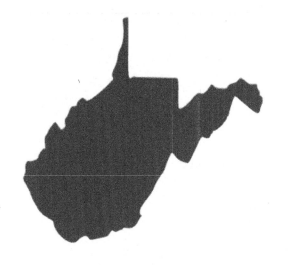

13.
- MASSACHUSETTS
- WEST VIRGINIA
- MINNESOTA
- VIRGINIA

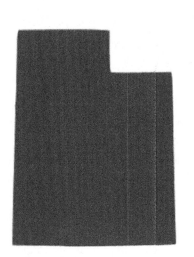

14.
- NORTH DAKOTA
- COLORADO
- KANSAS
- UTAH

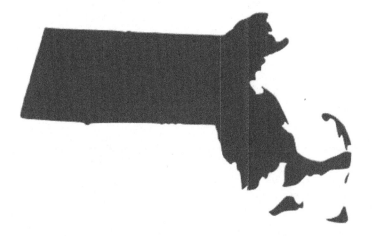

15.
- MASSACHUSETTS
- KENTUCKY
- RHODE ISLAND
- LOUISIANA

ANSWERS
STATE BIRDS, LANDMARKS, CAPITALS, FLAGS & MORE

DO YOU RECOGNIZE THE STATE? Name the state.

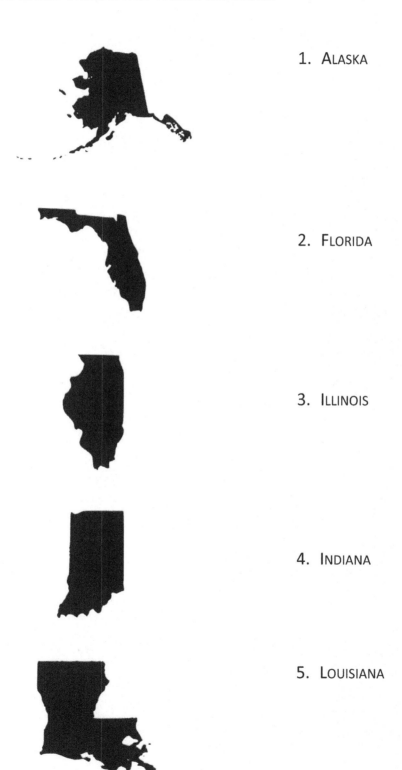

1. ALASKA

2. FLORIDA

3. ILLINOIS

4. INDIANA

5. LOUISIANA

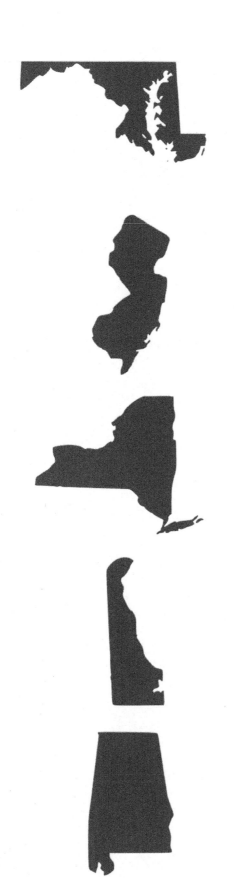

6. MARYLAND

7. NEW JERSEY

8. NEW YORK

9. DELAWARE

10. ALABAMA

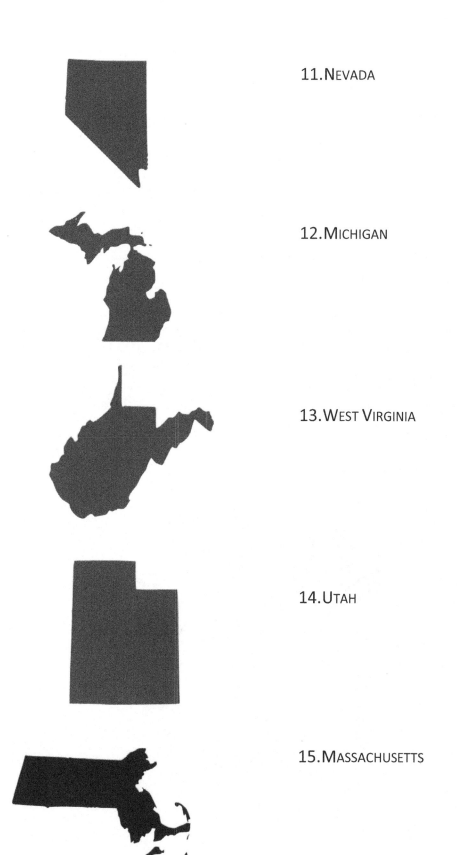

11. NEVADA

12. MICHIGAN

13. WEST VIRGINIA

14. UTAH

15. MASSACHUSETTS

ENTERTAINMENT & POP CULTURE

QUESTIONS 1 - 50
ENTERTAINMENT & POP CULTURE

1. What superhero first appeared during the 1940s? And can you describe the front cover?

2. Who were the Original Avengers in comics? (They were 5)

3. When did Captain America became an Avenger?

4. Which is the longest-running news television program? It is still on today, though the current format bears little resemblance to the debut episode on November 6, 1947.

5. What 1942 Best Picture winner famously contained the lines "Here's looking at you, kid" and "Play it, Sam. Play 'As Time Goes By'."?

6. And which actor said the phrase "Here's Looking at You, Kid"?

7. What was the first military-oriented film that Bud Abbott and Lou Costello starred in?

8. The 1940 classic "The Grapes of Wrath" featured a character by the name of Tom Joad. Who played the role of Tom Joad?

9. In the "Great Dictator" of 1940, Charlie Chaplin plays the role of a Jewish barber and also the role of the dictator of Tomania. What is the name of the dictator?

10. Do you know who Marion Morrison was? Tip: He met Wyatt Earp when he was just a prop boy in a Hollywood set.

11. What dark-haired Canadian Hollywood actress spent time in jail due to immigration-related problems, advanced from the chorus line to play Moses' wife in a movie epic, dated a real prince, and achieved her greatest popularity as Lily in the CBS television sitcom "The Munsters"?

12. Margarita Carmen Cansino was a big screen idol and the ultimate femme fatale from the 1940s. Referred to as the "Goddess of Love" she is best known for her performance in the movie "Gilda" (1946). What's her Hollywood name?

13. A type of light entertainment popular chiefly in the US from the mid1890s until the early 1930s, featuring a mixture of 10 to 15 individual unrelated acts featuring magicians, acrobats, comedians, trained animals, jugglers, singers, and dancers.

14. How did Judy Garland get her name?

15. In what movie did actress Natalie Wood debut in 1947 when she was just a child?

16. What is the name of the Hollywood Era that started during the Great Depression in the late 1920s and continued through to the early 1960s?

17. This actor who escaped at 10 years old to join a touring comedy troupe after his father's abandonment and the death of his mom (he later found out she wasn't dead but admitted in a psychiatric institution) was offered the role of James Bond but refused.

18. Name the five major studios during the Golden Era of Hollywood.

19. What was the first Technicolor movie?

20. What is a Canadian tuxedo and how did it come to be?

21. Which actor, from the Golden age of Hollywood, was known as 'The King of Hollywood'?

22. Who was Hollywood's first "It" girl? Tip: Her nickname was "Brooklyn Bonfire".

23. This type of swimsuit went for sale for the first time in Paris in 1946. What was it?

24. Which actress had twice the normal number of eyelashes and had MGM pay for her first wedding?

25. What awards, bestowed by the Hollywood Foreign Press Association, were held for the first time in 1944?

26. Which actor had his two front teeth knocked out while swinging on a trapeze in his aunt and uncle's barn. (He later embellished the story, saying he lost them in a motorcycle accident.)

27. Which actor was paid a record $3.7 million plus 12% of the gross profits for just 13 days work on Superman?

28. "Scarface" was the childhood nickname of this actor/singer who was a member of the "Rat Pack", a group that ruled the Las Vegas scene and performed on stage and in films of the early 1960s. Tip: He was known as "Ol' Blue Eyes".

29. Name the singer who in the mid-1940s found himself in the same lineup as a boisterous young comic at New York's Glass Hat Club. The kid's name was Jerry.

30. Which musician got his first job ever selling peanuts at Washington Senators games? Later, he became a famous American jazz pianist, composer, and leader of his eponymous jazz orchestra from 1923 through the rest of his life. Tip: His most famous song refers to a subway line in New York City.

31. Her family was very athletic. Her dad won three Olympic gold medals for sculling. Her mother was the coach of the women's team at the University of Pennsylvania. And her uncle won the Pulitzer Prize. Who is this actress? Tip: She married a prince.

32. This book, first published in 1946, is the 7th biggest seller of all time according to "The Top 10 of Everything" by Russell Ash (Hamlyn, 2008). It has sold over 50 million copies. Which book is it?

33. In 1947 this golfer, a former Olympic gold medalist, won the British Open for the first time, and in a career of more than 20 years won an astounding 82 tournaments in all. Who was it?

34. She's a member of the EGOT Club. (Emmy, Grammy, Oscar, and Tony awards). Tip: She won her Oscar for a movie based on the affair Princess Margaret had with commoner Peter Townsend.

35. What was the name of Lucy's neighbor and friend in "I Love Lucy"?

36. What did they do for a living?

37. Name the famous movie director who hosted a popular half-hour anthology television series featuring dramas, thrillers, mysteries and even horror? Tip: The program's theme music was Charles Gounod's "Funeral March of a Marionette".

38. How much was the first Polaroid Camera sold for in 1949?

39. What company began production of Italian sports cars in 1947?

40. In 1947, the world's first general purpose electronic computer, ENIAC, is completed, what does ENIAC stand for?

41. What was the name of the ranch in Bonanza?

42. Name the TV crime drama headed by Elliot Ness.

43. Name the actor that played Elliot Ness.

44. In 1955 an amusement park was opened in California, what was it called?

45. Who did Marilyn Monroe marry in 1954?

46. In 1952 the longest running play opened in London; it was…

47. Why did Agatha Christie write The Mousetrap?

48. Which company first introduced "TV Dinners" in 1954?

49. Four days after he was killed in a car crash, the film "Rebel Without a Cause" was released. Who was he?

50. What movie was James Dean filming when he died?

ANSWERS 1 - 50
ENTERTAINMENT & POP CULTURE

1. Captain America

This comic-strip superhero was created by writer Joe Simon and artist Jack Kirby for Timely (later Marvel) Comics. He debuted in March 1941 in Captain America Comics no. 1. The front cover showed Cap punching Nazi leader Adolf Hitler. It sold nearly one million copies.

2. The original Avengers consisted of Iron Man, Ant-Man, Hulk, Thor and the Wasp.

The team made its debut in The Avengers #1 (cover dated September 1963), created by writer-editor Stan Lee and artist/co-plotter Jack Kirby. Labeled "Earth's Mightiest Heroes".

3. Captain America was discovered trapped in ice in issue #4 and joined the group after they revived him.

4. Meet the Press

Meet the Press began as a radio show in 1945 and was reworked for television in 1947. It is currently the longest-running show on TV and has had 12 moderators in its history. Originally, it was a press conference-style show in which a newsmaker would take questions from a panel of journalists for 30 minutes.

5. Casablanca

Undeniably one of the highest regarded films of the 1940s Casablanca's legacy is nearly insurmountable including the quotes listed in the question, Casablanca has six quotes on The American Film Institute's list of the 100 greatest movie quotes of all time.

6. Humphrey Bogart

His line during the flashback scenes of Rick and Ilsa falling in love went on to become one of the most romantic dialogues in movie history

7. Buck Privates

When Universal Studios selected Bud Abbott and Lou Costello to headline "Buck Privates" in 1941, they had only appeared briefly in one other film. They proved to be box office leaders for years to come. The release was months before the United States entered WWII.

8. Henry Fonda

Henry Fonda was nominated for an Academy Award for Best Actor for his role as Tom Joad. However, he lost to James Stewart in the "Philadelphia Story". His first acting coach was Dorothy Brando, the mother of Marlon Brando

9. Adenoid Hynkel

This was Chaplin's first talking movie. However, he had made his name on the silent screen. He directed, produced, wrote, and acted in the movie.

Chaplin plays the roles of a Jewish barber and Hynkel, the dictator of Tomania. Hynkel orders all Jews to be captured but the barber escapes dressed as Hynkel. While out duck shooting and dressed as civilian, Hynkel is mistaken for the escaped barber and is imprisoned. The barber dressed as Hynkel addresses his followers and informs them that he (Hynkel) has changed his mind and wishes goodwill to all.
Chaplin later regretted doing the movie when he became aware of the persecution and horrors of concentration camps.

10. John Wayne

John Wayne's name was really Marion. If you think that name sounds a little funny for a big tough cowboy like Wayne, you aren't the only one. Terribly insecure, Marion Morrison utterly despised his feminine name. He was ready to jump on any other name that came along.

11. Yvonne De Carlo

Her best-known film roles were Anna Marie in Salome Where She Danced (1945); Anna in Criss Cross (1949); Sephora the wife of Moses in The Ten Commandments (1956), starring Charlton Heston; and Amantha Starr in Band of Angels (1957) with Clark Gable. In the early 1960s, De Carlo accepted the offer to play Lily Munster for the CBS television series The Munsters, alongside Fred Gwynne and Al Lewis.
While Prince Abdul Reza Pahlavi of Iran was visiting Hollywood, he met and became infatuated with De Carlo. Soon enough, he was sweeping her off her feet, even taking her to his royal palace in Tehran.

12. Rita Hayworth

Her parents were Spanish-born Eduardo Cansino who was a dancer, and her mother, Volga, who had been a Ziegfeld Follies. Soon after their daughter was born, they shortened her name to Rita Cansino. By the time Hayworth was 12, she was dancing professionally.

13. Vaudeville – A farce with music.

American Vaudeville, more so than any other mass entertainment, grew out of the culture of incorporation that defined American life after the Civil War. The development of vaudeville marked the beginning of popular entertainment as big business, dependent on the organizational efforts of a growing number of white-collar workers and the increased leisure time, spending power, and changing tastes of an urban middle class audience.

14. Originally, Judy was Frances Gumm. Judy and her sisters, toured the vaudeville circuit as "The Gumm Sisters" for many years. In 1934 they were encouraged to choose a more appealing name after "Gumm" was met with laughter from the audience. They changed their name to "The Garland Sisters".

One year later, in 1935, "Frances Garland" changed her first name to Judy, after the popular song "Judy" by *Hoagy Carmichael*, to become Judy Garland.

15. In the classic holiday film "Miracle on 34th Street" (1947).

She played Susana Walker, a cynical girl who comes to believe a kindly department store holiday season employee portrayed by Edmund Gwenn is the real Santa Claus. The film has become a Christmas classic.

She was counted among the top child stars in Hollywood after the film and was so popular that Macy's invited her to appear in the store's annual Thanksgiving Day Parade.

16. The Golden Age of Hollywood.

It was a period in American filmmaking in which the five major studios dominated the production of major pictures, controlling every aspect of a film's production, from casting to shooting to distribution, even having celebrities sign extremely strict contracts.

17. Cary Grant, whose real name was Archibald Leach.

Grant was close friends with Bond producer Albert "Cubby" Broccoli; he was even best man at Broccoli's wedding. Their relationship made it inevitable Broccoli would offer him the role. It was ideal casting, but two things hindered the deal. For one, Grant refused to commit to a multi-picture contract, as was eventually required of Sean Connery. For another, Grant was already 58 years old. So, he passed.

18. MGM, Paramount, Fox, Warner Bros, and RKO.

The golden age of Hollywood was a period in American filmmaking in which the five major studios dominated the production of major motion pictures, controlling every aspect of a film's production, from casting to shooting to distribution.

The golden age relied on "stars" such as Humphrey Bogart, Cary Grant, Grace Kelly, and Rita Hayworth, to carry its films to success at the box office. Although there's some contention as to when the golden age began and ended, most critics agree that it "existed" in some capacity from the late 1910s into the early 1960s.

19. The first Technicolor film shot entirely in Technicolor's three-color process was "Becky Sharp" in 1935.

Later, there were two movies that changed everything for color in film: The Wizard of Oz and Snow White and the Seven Dwarfs.

20. Think of a Canadian tuxedo as any denim-on-denim look. Denim shirt and jeans would be the perfect Canadian tux. Denim dress and matching boots? That's also a (slightly fancier) Canadian tux.

Legend has it that back in 1951, singer Bing Crosby wasn't permitted to check into a high-end hotel in Vancouver because he was wearing, you guessed it, a denim-on-denim outfit (before denim-on-denim was certified fashion trend it was considered a sartorial faux pas). Word traveled fast, and in no time at all, denim giant Levi's designed him a custom tuxedo that was made entirely out of denim. Just like that, a cultural icon was born!

21. For many years, the Hollywood press dubbed Clark Gable as" The King".

Born and raised in Ohio, Gable traveled to Hollywood where he began his film career as an extra in silent films between 1924 and 1926. He progressed to supporting roles for Metro-Goldwyn-Mayer, and his first leading role in Dance, Fools, Dance (1931) was alongside Joan Crawford, who requested him for the part. He had roles in more than 60 motion pictures in multiple genres during a career that lasted 37 years, three decades of which was as a leading man. Gable died of a heart attack at the age of 59; his final on-screen appearance was as an aging cowboy in The Misfits, released posthumously in 1961.

22. Clara Bow

She rose to stardom during the silent film era of the 1920s and successfully made the transition to "talkies" in 1929. Her appearance as a plucky shopgirl in the film "It" brought her global fame and the nickname "The It Girl".

Definition of "It":
That quality possessed by some which draws all others with its magnetic force. With 'It' you win all men if you are a woman and all women if you are a man. 'It' can be a quality of the mind as well as a physical attraction.

23. Bikini

On July 5, 1946, French designer Louis Réard unveils a daring two-piece swimsuit at the Piscine Molitor, a popular swimming pool in Paris.

Parisian showgirl Micheline Bernardini modeled the new fashion, which Réard dubbed "bikini," inspired by a news-making U.S. atomic test that took place off the Bikini Atoll in the Pacific Ocean earlier that week.

24. Elizabeth Taylor

While most women enhance their eyelash line with mascara and falsies, Taylor didn't have to. She had genetic mutation known as Lymphedema-distichiasis syndrome. Apparently, 7 percent of people with this mutation also have congenital heart disease, and Taylor did have heart troubles that led to her death.

When Taylor married Conrad Hilton Jr. in 1950, her film career had taken off and he had a sizable fortune due to his father's hotel chain. Though neither of them would have struggled to pay for their 600-guest affair, Metro-Goldwyn-Mayer actually paid for the whole thing.

25. The Golden Globe Awards

The first Golden Globe Awards, honoring the best achievements in 1943 filmmaking, were held late on January 20, 1944, at the 20th Century Fox studios in Los Angeles, California.

26. James Dean

As an adult, he purportedly enjoyed surprising acquaintances by casually removing his false teeth mid-conversation.

27. Marlon Brando

Back on June 30, 1976, it was reported that Marlon Brando agreed to play the title character's father in "Superman" for a salary that was "unprecedented." It was eventually revealed that the actor was paid $3.7 million and an amazing 11.75% backend to play Jor-El, for 13 days work and less than 20 minutes onscreen. In comparison, Christopher Reeve earned $250,000 in the title role, dominating most of the 143-minute running time.

28. Frank Sinatra

After his professional career had stalled by the early 1950s, Sinatra turned to Las Vegas where he became one of the scene's prominent pioneer performers and the eventual leader of the Rat Pack, after the death of its original leader Humphrey Bogart.

He was also called Scarface as a child due to scarring on his face from birth.

When Frank Sinatra was born on December 12, 1915, everybody thought he was stillborn. He was a huge baby, at 13.5 pounds, and the doctors had removed him from the womb with forceps.

His grandmother ran him under some cold water in the kitchen sink and low and behold, little Francis Albert was actually alive. However, the forceps left severe scarring on his left cheek, neck, and permanently damaged his ear.

29. Dean Martin

Dean Martin and Jerry Lewis formed the most electric comedy team in the history of show business. Joining together in the summer of 1946, their act caught on like wildfire.

30. Duke Ellington

Composer, conductor, and entertainer amid the Harlem Renaissance. During the developmental Cotton Club years, he explored different avenues regarding and built up the style that would rapidly bring him overall achievement.

"Take the 'A' Train" was composed in 1939 by Billy Strayhorn after Ellington offered Strayhorn a job in his organization and gave him money to travel from Pittsburgh to New York City. Ellington wrote directions for Strayhorn to get to his house by subway, directions that began, "Take the A Train".

31. Grace Kelly

Grace's brother was also a rowing champion and won the bronze medal in the 1956 Olympic Games. This princess came from a talented family.

32. "The Common Sense Book of Baby and Child Care" by Dr. Benjamin Spock

Dr. Spock, not to be confused with Mr. Spock, had the revolutionary idea that parents should trust their own common sense because "you know more than you think." He was blamed by some that this concept led to the self-indulgence of the flower power generation of the 1960s.

33. Babe Didrikson Zaharias

Mildred "Babe" Didrikson won gold medals at the 1932 Los Angeles Olympics in the javelin, high jump and hurdles. She was the first woman to compete in a men's golf tournament, something no other woman even tried for more than half a century. In 1938 she married wrestler George Zaharias and died of cancer in 1956.

34. Audrey Hepburn

One of 14 people in the world, she's won an Emmy (hosting Gardens of the World with Audrey Hepburn), a Grammy (spoken word album Audrey Hepburn's Enchanted Tales), an Oscar (best actress in Roman Holiday), and a Tony (best actress in Ondine).

35. Ethel (Ethel and Fred Mertz)

36. To survive, the couple worked at a diner, Fred as the waiter and Ethel as the cook.

It is likely that they were in vaudeville together the first five years of their marriage, as Ethel once says (before her California trip) that she hadn't been out of New York for 20 out of the 25 years she had been married.

37. Alfred Hitchcock

Alfred Hitchcock Presents premiered on October 2, 1955. Originally running at half an hour, the show was later extended to a full hour and retitled The Alfred Hitchcock Hour. Despite what the viewer may be led to believe, Hitchcock only directed 17 of the 268 filmed episodes.

38. $89.95

If we adjust that amount to December 2021 dollars, it will equal around $1,530. That's right: a brand-new Polaroid camera would have cost about the same as a premium model iPhone.

39. Ferrari

The company officially launched in 1947. However, the automaker's legendary founder and namesake Enzo Ferrari was involved in the industry long before then.

40. Electronic Numerical Integrator Analyzer and Computer

It was the first programmable, electronic, general-purpose digital computer, completed in 1945. There were other computers that had these features, but the ENIAC had all of them in one package. It was Turing-complete and able to solve "a large class of numerical problems" through reprogramming.

41. Ponderosa

The Ponderosa was the fictional setting for Bonanza. According to the 9th episode ("Mr. Henry Comstock") in the first season, it was a thousand-square mile (640,000 acre or 2,600 km²) ranch on the shores of Lake Tahoe, nestled high in the Sierra Nevada, with a large ranch house in the center of it.

The inspiration for the name was the large number of Ponderosa pines, which grow above 5,000-foot altitude, in the fictional ranch's location. A Latin derivation would be large (root of the English word ponderous).

42. The Untouchables

43.Robert Stack

Fun fact. Elliot Ness met Al Capone just once.

On May 3, 1932, Ness was among the federal agents who took Capone from the Cook County Jail to Dearborn Station, where he boarded the Dixie Flyer to the Atlanta Federal Penitentiary; the only time the two men are known to have met in person.

44. Disneyland

The opening of Disneyland was televised by the ABC network. The hosts of the broadcast were Ronald Reagan, Art Linkletter, and Bob Cummings. The estimated TV audience was around 90 million, an incredible high number given the fact that not everyone in America had television sets in those days. The general admission that year was ONE U.S. dollar per entrant.

45. Joe DiMaggio

Joe DiMaggio, one of the greatest baseball players of all time, married Hollywood starlet Marilyn Monroe on Jan. 14, 1954. The pair were wed in a private ceremony at San Francisco City Hall. DiMaggio first sought out Monroe after seeing a picture of her posing with White Sox outfielder Gus Zernial in 1951.

46. The Mousetrap

Agatha Christie's The Mousetrap is the longest running show, of any kind, in the world. It opened in November 1952 at The Ambassadors Theatre in London and moved to St. Martin's Theatre in March 1974 where it is still running to this day.

47. The Mousetrap was originally written as a 20-minute radio drama for Queen Mary as an 80th birthday gift, following Queen Mary's request for a new radio play by Christie.

48. Swanson

By 1954, Quaker State Foods had produced and sold over 2,500,000 frozen dinners! The concept really took hold in 1954 when Swanson's frozen meals appeared. Swanson was a well-known brand that consumers recognized, and Swanson launched a massive advertising campaign for their product.

49. James Dean

At 5:45 PM on September 30, 1955, 24-year-old actor James Dean is killed in Cholame, California, when the Porsche he is driving hits a Ford Tudor sedan at an intersection. The driver of the other car, 23-year-old California Polytechnic State University student Donald Turnupseed, was dazed but mostly uninjured; Dean's passenger, German Porsche mechanic Rolf Wütherich was badly injured but survived.

50. Giant

James Dean's best friend voiced one scene in Giant after his tragic death. At the time of Dean's death, he had just finished filming for the movie Giant, but the production wasn't yet complete.

51. Which popular fast food chain restaurant featuring only hamburgers, potato chips (later replaced by french fries), drinks, and pie was first opened in 1955?

52. What popular toy was first introduced by Wham-O in 1958?

53. Charlie Brown is noted for two features. One is his sweater with the oversized tooth pattern which he almost always wears. The other is something that he was often teased about. Which one is it?

54. This **comedy** featuring the home life of a **Jewish** family, supposedly located at 1038 East Tremont Avenue in **the Bronx airs live on CBS in 1949 as one of the very first** television sitcoms.

55. Name Elvis Presley's first film.

57. What was DuMont?

58. Which American television sitcom, starring Lucille Ball and Desi Arnaz was released on 15 October 1951?

59. The title of the bestselling book of 1951 came from a Rudyard Kipling poem. The plot centers on a group of Army officers and the women in their lives in Hawaii just before the bombing of Pearl Harbor. Which James Jones novel is this?

60. In 1950, Peanuts, a syndicated daily and Sunday American comic strip appeared. Who was the writer and illustrator?

61. Do you remember the name of the first Peanuts comic strip?

62. This first book of a trilogy by an author born in South Africa (but who considered himself English/British) first appeared in 1954. Tip: These books were considered the first fantasy books. They were turn into movies by director Peter Jackson.

63. The first episode of a long-running family saga appeared in 1952. The sitcom involved two sons, one of whom was a "rock star" who died (in real life) in a plane crash in 1985. What television show was this?

64. What film, from 1956, with a character named "Passepartout", played by the actor Cantinflas and based on a novel by Jules Verne, came first in the contest for the Oscar Award for Best Picture?

65. What children's book by Theodore Geisel, which spawned a movie starring Mike Myers in 2003, was first published in 1957?

66. Who was the original host of "Meet the Press"?

67. By what name was NBC News previously known?

68. Who was the original host of the "Today" show?

69. Do you remember his famous signoff?

70. Who was the "Today" show's famous non-human cohost?

71. Which American humor magazine first published in 1952 often featured its mascot, Alfred E. Neuman, on the cover with his face replacing that of a celebrity or character who was being lampooned?

72. What was the name of the Hollywood production facility opened by CBS in 1952?

73. What was the first television series to be regularly broadcast in color?

74. What was the answer to the question: "Say kids, what time is it?"

75. From 1950 until 1959 which of the following television shows was not ranked number one for a given year?

76. Which famous rock and roll artist was known to his fans as "The King"?

77. Where did Fats Domino find his thrill?

78. Which chain of discount department stores first opened in Garden City, Michigan in 1962? Tip: Its original name was S.S. Kresge Co.

79. What Queen song lasts nearly 6 minutes, 3 minutes longer than most songs that received radio airplay? It said it would never sell.

80. Which of these '60s bands sang "California Dreamin"?

81. Who was the lead singer of the Doors in the 1960s?

82. From which sci-fi television show comes the phrase "Live long and prosper" accompanied by a formal hand gesture.? The (lesser known) response is "Peace and long life.

83. What safety device did Allen Breed invent in 1968?

84. Can you name the drummer of the Beatles?

85. The first VCR home video recorder was introduced by what company in 1964?

86. What is Elton John's real name?

87. Which nickname does the vocalist and bass player of the Police, Gordon Summer, go by?

88. Can you name the country star known to his fans as "The Man in Black"?

89. Who died alongside J.P. "The Big Bopper" Richardson and Ritchie Valens in a plane crash on February 3, 1959?

90. What rebellious form of music gained traction in the 1970s?

91. What does the phrase from a famous song "The day the music died" refers to? Who wrote this famous song and what is the name of it?

92. The second to last line of the opening theme song of this comedy sitcom was "Gee, our old LaSalle ran great"? What's the name of this show?

93. True or false? The term "rock and roll" was first used to describe a musical genre by disc jockey Alan Freed.

94. Can you name the massive music festival that began on August 5, 1969?

95. Which groovy '70s fad that used the same technology as some of our favorite modern-day devices could tell the mood?

96. Starting in 1970, a cheerful bright yellow symbol started showing up on buttons, mugs, and t-shirts. What was the four-word expression often depicted with this smiling image?

97. Which popular car in the '70s was used in the movie "The Italian Job"?

98. What major law was violated in the movie Smokey and the Bandit?

99. What was Rizzo's real name in Grease?

100. Which relative of John Travolta's made a cameo appearance in Saturday Night Fever?

51. McDonald's

The first McDonald's restaurant was opened in 1940 by brothers Maurice and Richard McDonald in San Bernardino, California. It originally was a drive-in that offered a wide selection of items. However, in 1948 the brothers changed to a simple and efficient format that they named the Speedee Service System.

This included a self-service counter where customers received their food quickly because hamburgers were cooked ahead of time, wrapped, and warmed under heat lamps. These innovations allowed the brothers to charge just 15 cents for a basic hamburger, about half the price of competing restaurants. McDonald's was a huge success, and the brothers began a franchise program.

Appliances for McDonald's were purchased from a salesman named Ray Kroc, who was intrigued by their need for eight malt and shake mixers. In 1954 he visited the restaurant to see how a small shop could sell so many milk shakes.

Kroc became a franchise agent for the brothers. In April 1955 Kroc launched McDonald's Systems, Inc., later known as McDonald's Corporation. In 1961 Kroc bought out the McDonald brothers.

52. The Hula Hoop

The Hula-Hoop, a hip-swiveling toy that became a huge fad across America when it was first marketed by Wham-O in 1958, was patented by the company's co-founder, Arthur "Spud" Melin.

An estimated 25 million Hula-Hoops were sold in its first four months of production alone.

53. His large head.

His sister is Sally, three years younger than Charlie; Snoopy is indeed his dog, and his favorite baseball player is Joe Schalbotnik. But it's his oversized head that he is tormented for: "Is that the Moon? No, it's just Charlie Brown's head!" It's also mentioned in "It's the Great Pumpkin, Charlie Brown!".

54. The Goldbergs

It is a comedy-drama broadcast from 1929 to 1946 on American radio, and from 1949 to 1956 on American television. It was adapted into a 1948 play, Me and Molly; a 1950 film The Goldbergs, and a 1973 Broadway musical, Molly.

55. Love Me Tender

It is an American black and white Western about for brothers, the Renos. It was the only time in his entire career that he was not billed as the lead.

57. A TV network.

DuMont, the 'fourth network', was unable to compete with NBC, CBS and ABC and ceased operations in 1956.

58. I Love Lucy

"I Love Lucy", a hundred laughs a minute, stars Lucille Ball who plays the part of Lucy, a dippy woman who constantly strives to become a star along with her Bandleader husband, played by Desi Arnaz.

59. From Here to Eternity

James Jones won the National Book Award for "From Here to Eternity." The reference to the book's title is from Kipling's poem "Gentleman-rankers" which ends with the verse: "We're poor little lambs who've lost our way, Baa! Baa! Baa! We're little black sheep who've gone astray, Baa--aa--aa! Gentlemen-rankers out on the spree, damned from here to Eternity, God ha' mercy on such as we, Baa! Yah! Bah!"

60. It was written and illustrated by Charles M. Schulz. The strip's original run extended from 1950 to 2000, continuing in reruns afterward.

61. The first Peanuts comic strip, and the first time Charlie Brown is called, "Good ol' Charlie Brown".

62. The Fellowship of the Ring

"The Hobbit" (Otherwise known as "There and Back Again") was published in 1937, seventeen years before the "official" initial book in the "Lord of the Rings" trilogy was written. Hardly anyone would deny that Tolkien was the ultimate "first" in the fantasy epic genre.

63. The Adventures of Ozzie and Harriet

"The Adventures of Ozzie and Harriet" was the longest running sitcom in the U.S. history until it was overtaken by "The Simpsons" in 2004. Teen idol Ricky Nelson went on to have hits such as "Traveling Man", "Hello, Mary Lou", and "Garden Party".

64. Around the World in 80 Days

This film starred David Niven as Phileas Fogg who, on a bet, travelled around the world using various methods of transportation, but most notably in a balloon. In the Spanish version of the movie, Cantinflas was billed as the starring actor. Regardless, with the help of the acting abilities of Shirley MacLaine, this movie made it to number one in 1956.

65. The Cat in the Hat

Theodore Geisel is the birth name of the author Dr. Seuss. After "The Cat in the Hat" was written, it became a "first reader" in many primary/elementary schools in North America, replacing the overly simplified (and perhaps boring for young imaginative minds) "Dick and Jane" and (Spot) stories.

66. Martha Rountree

While Rountree was the original commentator, it was "American Mercury Magazine" editor, Lawrence Spivak who anchored the popular news program for almost thirty years. Spivak was the host from 1974 to 1975 when his last guest was President Gerald R. Ford, the first incumbent President to appear.

67. Camel Newsreel Theatre

Camel Newsreel Theatre, sponsored by Camel cigarettes, began as a ten-minute long Movietone Newsreels show featuring John Cameron Swayze. It later expanded to fifteen minutes and Swayze narrated the news.

68. Dave Garroway

He was joined by Jack Lescoulie, who did sports and Jim Fleming reading the news. From its beginning, a glass window viewing he New York streets was a part of the set, a tradition which survives until today.

69. Peace

70. J. Fred Muggs

The show's early ratings were not promising, and the producers wanted to make the show more entertaining. They added a chimpanzee named J. Fred Muggs, who became an almost instant popular star in his own right.

71. Mad (stylized as MAD)

No one really knows where Alfred came from. Before MAD put him on the cover of their issue #21, his likeness could be traced to other characters all the way back to the 1890s, such as The Yellow Kid (from the comic strip Hogan's alley of Richard F. Outcault fame). Harvey Kurtzman, founder of MAD, claims he spotted Alfred on a postcard and named him after composer Alfred Neuman.

72. Television City

Before CBS's move, most television shows originated from New York or Chicago. Afterwards, the other networks began moving to the Los Angeles area.

73. The Colgate Comedy Hour

The variety show featured top-named entertainers and was broadcast live from New York. The November 22, 1953, show was hosted by Donald O'Connor and was the very first color TV broadcast.

74. It's Howdy Doody Time!

Most American "baby boomers" grew up watching the 27-inch marionette and his human companion "Buffalo" Smith and their adventures in Doodyville.

75. Dragnet

The Jack Webb production, "Dragnet" was in the top 10 shows for most of the decade of the 50s, but only reached as high as number two in the 1953-54 season behind "I Love Lucy".

76. Elvis Presley

Without a doubt the most famous name in rock and roll, Elvis Presley first came to prominence in the mid-1950s. His career spanned three different decades and included his "comeback" in the late '60s, after a period of inactivity, when Elvis began performing in Las Vegas. Sadly, Presley died of a heart attack in 1977. He was only 42.

77. On Blueberry Hill

Fats Domino released his version of "Blueberry Hill" in 1956, and it reached No. 2 on the Billboard Hot 100 and No. 1 on the R&B charts. But did you know the song was actually first released in 1940 and recorded many times before Fats Domino, by artists including the Glen Miller Orchestra and Gene Autry.

78. Kmart

When the first Kmart discount store opened on March 1, 1962, in Garden City, Michigan, 4000 curious customers waited in line for the doors to finally unlock. Kresge intended for Kmart to have a national presence. By the end of 1962, 18 Kmarts were in operation. Within a decade, that number swelled to 800.

79. Bohemian Rhapsody

But it did sell - over one million copies in just three months. It also stayed at No. 1 on the British charts for nine weeks and to date remains Queen's top-selling single.

80. The Mamas and the Papas

The song "California Dreamin'" has been recorded by many artists. Originally written by John and Michelle Phillips, it is their version with the Mamas and the Papas that is the best known.

81. Jim Morrison

The Doors were extremely successful in the late 1960s. Their lead singer, Jim Morrison, was also the band's chief songwriter. He is regarded by many as one of rock music's greatest front man. Morrison died at the age of 27.

82. Star Trek

The Vulcan "salute" was devised by Leonard Nimoy, who portrayed the half Vulcan character Mr. Spock on the original Star Trek television series. A 1968 New York Times interview described the gesture as a "double-fingered version of Churchill's victory sign". Nimoy said in that interview that he "decided that the Vulcans were a 'hand-oriented' people".

In his 1975 autobiography I Am Not Spock, Nimoy, who was Jewish, wrote that he based it on the Priestly Blessing performed by Jewish Kohanim with both hands, thumb to thumb in this same position, representing the Hebrew letter Shin, which has three upward strokes like the position of the thumb and fingers in the gesture. Nimoy wrote that when he was a child, his grandfather took him to an Orthodox synagogue, where he saw the blessing performed and was impressed by it.

83. Automatic Airbag

Allen K. Breed is an inventor, entrepreneur, and pioneer in one of the most significant advances in automotive safety of recent times, the air bag.

84. Ringo Starr

Richard Starkey, or as the world knows him, Ringo Starr, is the drummer of the Beatles, possibly the greatest group of all time, despite the fact that they were only together for a decade. Interestingly, Starr was not the original drummer of the band and only joined them in 1962, replacing Pete Best.

85. Sony

The Sony Company took the idea that Ampex created and began to expand on the technology. In 1963, Sony created the first reel-to-reel recorder. This was innovative and the technology helped to make the machines less expensive for consumers, but they were still out of reach for the majority of households

86. Reginald Kenneth Dwight

With over 300 million records sold worldwide, Elton John, or is that Reginald Dwight, certainly doesn't need an introduction. John has been recording since the 1960s, writing songs in a partnership with lyricist Bernie Taupin.

87. Sting

Born in 1951, Gordon Sumner, or Sting as he is known, is the main songwriter, vocalist and bass player of the Police. He gained his nickname because he often wore a black-and-yellow-striped sweater that bandmates in the Phoenix Jazzmen, an early group he played in, said made him look like a bee. And the name Sting was born.

88. Johnny Cash

Johnny Cash recorded his first songs at the legendary Sun Records studio in Memphis, Tennessee, in 1955. In fact, at one point in those early years, Cash, Elvis Presley, Carl Perkins and Jerry Lee Lewis all happened to be in the studio together and jammed. This was recorded, with some of the songs surviving to this day.

89. Buddy Holly

An event that shocked the music world, the light aircraft crash on February 3, 1959, saw Buddy Holly, the up-and-coming Ritchie Valens and J.P. "The Big Bopper" Richardson all killed. The pilot, who lost control of the plane in bad weather, also died.

90. Punk

The punk movement exploded in the 1970s on both sides of the Atlantic. In the United States, bands such as the New York Dolls and the Ramones drove the movement, while in the United Kingdom, the Sex Pistols had early success.

91. Don McLean wrote the song "American Pie".

He famously referenced the death of Buddy Holly, J.P. "The Big Bopper" Richardson, and Ritchie Valens as "the day the music died".

92. All in the Family.

The show received a lot of calls and mail about the theme song. People had so much trouble understanding this line.

O'Connor and Stapleton re-recorded it prior to season three and carefully enunciated the mystery lyric. (The LaSalle was a high-end General Motors model that was manufactured from 1927 until 1940.)

93. True

Although rock and roll were a term heard in R&B songs from the 1930s, it was Alan Freed who first used it to describe a new musical genre. Early rock and roll artists included Big Joe Turner, who sang the song "Shake, Rattle & Roll."

94. Woodstock

Held on a dairy farm near Bethel in New York, Woodstock was a music festival billed as "An Aquarian Exposition: 3 Days of Peace & Music." It ran from August 15–18, 1969, and featured 32 artists, including Jimi Hendrix, Joan Baez, the Grateful Dead, Janis Joplin and the Who.

95. Mood Rings

Changing the channel back to the 1970s, the mood ring was a product of the "Me Decade," during which Americans embraced individualism over national and political interests for one of the first times in history. With no Facebook, Twitter, Instagram, or TikTok to broadcast oneself, people used the color-changing rings to wear their feelings on their fingers.

96. Have a Nice Day.

According to reports, the smiley face was originally designed by a graphic artist hired to create an image to raise employee morale for a large life insurance company. Though they put it on buttons and stickers to hand out to cheer people, they didn't Copywrite the image.

Years later, two Hallmark card shop owners in Philadelphia came across the buttons, added "Have a Nice Day" and—copywriting their revised version—made a mint while cheering up Americans everywhere.

97. A Mini Cooper

The film's plot centers around Cockney criminal Charlie Croker, recently released from prison, who forms a gang for the job of stealing a cache of gold bullion being transported through the city of Turin, Italy in an armored security truck.

98. Smuggling Coors beer east of the Mississippi.

Big Enos (Pat McCormick) wants to drink Coors at a truck show, but in 1977 it was illegal to sell Coors east of the Mississippi River without a permit. Truck driver Bo "Bandit" Darville (Burt Reynolds) agrees to pick up the beer in Texas and drive it to Georgia within 28 hours. When Bo picks up hitchhiker Carrie (Sally Field), he attracts the attention of Sheriff Buford T. Justice (Jackie Gleason). Angry that Carrie will not marry his son, Justice embarks on a high-speed chase after Bandit.

99. Betty

Stockard Channing (born Susan Antonia Williams Stockard; February 13, 1944) is an American actress. She is known for playing Betty Rizzo in the film Grease (1978) and First Lady Abbey Bartlet in the NBC television series The West Wing (1999–2006).

100. John Travolta's mother

She made the cameo appearance in the very beginning of the movie. She played the female customer to whom John Travolta gives a discount on paint in the paint store.

According to the credits on IMDb, also his sister Ann Travolta had a role. Her official role was the "Pizza Girl".

101. What was the name of the '70s toy that used colorful pegs and lights?

102. In Blazing Saddles, what is the last name of everybody in the town of Rock Ridge?

103. In Halloween, Michael Myers wore a Halloween mask of what famous character?

104. What was the name of Steven Spielberg's first hit movie which was released in 1975?

105. True success didn't come until after her death at age 27, with the posthumous album release of her last album titled "Pearl."

106. In 1966, Chas Chandler the bassist for The Animals, saw this musician playing at Cafe Wha? in New York City. He first thought "This guy doesn't seem anything special, then all of a sudden he started playing with his teeth,". Name this famous guitarist.

107. What television show that takes place during the Korean War was popular in the 1970s?

108. Who won a boxing match against George Foreman?

109. Which popular sketch-comedy series first aired in 1975 in New York?

110. What '70s children's television show featured a crew of round characters with large eyes?

111. In Texas Chainsaw Massacre, there was a guy in a wheelchair. What was his name?

112. In Animal House, what was Bluto's grade point average?

113. Which dolls, created in 1959, had a pet horse called Dancer? These dolls gained huge popularity in the 70s.

114. Who was the set dresser for Brian DePalma's Phantom of the Paradise?

115. What product released in the '70s allowed people to take music with them?

116. In Grease, who do we see first, the Pink Ladies or the T-Birds?

117. In the early 19th century, when a standardized uniform did not yet exist in the U.S. Navy, some sailors adopted a style of wide trousers ending in bell-shaped cuffs. What is the name of these trousers?

118. What character did Harrison Ford play in Star Wars?

119. Who was originally supposed to play Indiana Jones in "Raiders Of The Lost Ark"?

120. Seven people from different walks of life are cast away at an unknown island after a violent storm. What is the name of this show?

121. Which fighter was initially supposed to fight Apollo Creed in Rocky?

122. Which famous British rock band got the idea for their name from Buddy Holly and the Crickets?

123. Born LaDonna Adrian Gaines, she was known as the "Queen of Disco", while her music gained a global following during the disco era of the 1970s. What was her stage name?

124. What mesmerizing light fixture containing a viscous liquid in which a brightly colored waxy substance is suspended became very popular in the 70s?

125. The popular line "Leave the gun. Take the cannoli," comes from which movie?

126. Where do Lex Luthor and the villains find the meteorite that fell to Earth from Krypton?

127. In Superman, where does Miss Teschmacher's mother live?

128. What console was released in 1977?

129. Which toy from the '70s was filled with corn syrup?

130. The goal of this shoot 'em up arcade game developed by Tomohiro Nishikado in 1978 was to defeat wave after wave of descending aliens with a horizontally moving laser. What is the name of this video game?

131. Which rock icon died on August 16, 1977, in Memphis, Tennessee?

132. Do you recognize the following slogan? What show does it belong to?

"You are about to enter another dimension. A dimension not only of sight and sound but of mind. A journey into a wondrous land of imagination. Next stop..."

133. Why did Sandy become ill during the sleepover at Frenchy's house?

134. In 1972, the first U.S. cable subscription service was launched. What was the name of it?

135. What was the charter boat called on Gilligan's Island?

136. What was the dummy's name in Magic?

137. Who was the first African American to grace the cover of Vogue in 1973?

138. What type of shoes were fashionable in the '70s?

139. Which hairstyle was popular for women in the 1970s? Tip: It was Farrah Fawcett's hairstyle.

140. In 'Empire Strikes Back' when the ghost of Obi Wan Kenobi said that Luke was their last hope against the Empire, who was Yoda referring to when he said: "No, there is another"?

141. Which Atari video game, released in 1972, was the first one to have real commercial success? Tip: It was a simple-yet-fun and addictive game resembling an electronic tennis game.

142. This orange lasagna and pizza lover was created on June 19, 1978, by artist Jim Davis. Who is it?

143. What is the ship called in Alien 1979?

144. Astonishing the entire world with her 30-second perfect routine on the uneven bars, this gymnast was awarded the first 10 in the history of Olympic gymnastics competitions.

145. What singer/songwriter appeared in the film Two Lane Blacktop?

146. What was the dog's name in Smokey and The Bandit?

147. On August 1, 1981, what famous cable TV channel dedicated to music made its debut?

148. What was the very first James Bond movie that was shown in the 80's? What was the last?

149. Name the actress who played the pretty blond girl Elliot danced with in E.T. The Extra-Terrestrial?

150. In 1982, what famous Disney World Park (from its initials Experimental Prototype Community of Tomorrow) opened?

ENTERTAINMENT & POP CULTURE

101. The Lite-Brite

The Lite-Brite was a must-have toy in the '70s. Kids could make pictures or words using the colored pegs that could be stuck into the main light box.

102. Johnson

It's 1874 in the American frontier of the wild west. Because of geological problems, a railroad under construction needs to be rerouted through the town of Rock Ridge, a frontier town where everyone has the last name of "Johnson" (including a "Howard Johnson", a "Dr. Samuel Johnson", a "Van Johnson" and an "Olson N. Johnson").

103. He wore a Captain Kirk (Star Trek) mask that was painted white.

Michael Myers' legendarily terrifying mask in the original Halloween is actually an altered Captain Kirk mask that production designer and editor Lee Wallace bought for a couple of bucks at a random store on Hollywood Boulevard and it ended up being used in the movie.

104. Jaws

Steven Spielberg's first true hit movie was "Jaws," which was released in 1975. The movie is now regarded as one of the best of all time.

Spielberg may be one of the biggest directors ever now, but back when the production for "Jaws" began he only had one feature to his name, "The Sugarland Express." Producers initially offered the job to Rick Richards. However, for some weird reason Richards kept calling the shark in the movie a "whale," and producers dropped him and replaced him with Spielberg.

105. Janis Joplin

She was still working on "Pearl" when she died, meaning producer Paul Rothchild had to finish the project without her.

In 1967, Joplin rose to fame following an appearance at Monterey Pop Festival, where she was the lead singer of the then little-known San Francisco psychedelic rock band Big Brother and the Holding Company. After releasing two albums with the band, she left Big Brother to continue as a solo artist.

Five singles by Joplin reached the *Billboard* Hot 100, including a cover of the Kris Kristofferson song "Me and Bobby McGee", which reached number one in March 1971. Her most popular songs include her cover versions of "Piece of My Heart", "Cry Baby", "Down on Me", "Ball and Chain", "Summertime", and her original song "Mercedes Benz", her final recording.

106. Jimi Hendrix

Chas Chandler became Jimi's manager. When they met Hendrix was performing as Jimmy James and it was Chandler who suggested he use the name "Jimi."

107. M*A*S*H

M*A*S*H was a very popular television show in the '70s. It took place during the Korean War and revolved around the nurses and doctors who took care of the casualties.

108. Muhammad Ali

Muhammad Ali knocked out George Foreman in the historic boxing match known as 'Rumble in the Jungle.'

109. Saturday Night Live.

The series began, in part, because Johnny Carson wanted more time off from his late-night show.

Do you remember its iconic intro line? "Live from New York, it's Saturday night!". During the show's first episode, Chevy Chase had the honor of saying the iconic intro line.

110. The Flumps

The adventures of a family of cute, furry creatures. They were Grandpa Flump, Ma and Pa Flump, their eldest son Perkin, daughter Posie and youngest son Pootle.

111. Franklin

He is Sally Hardesty's invalidated brother that suffers from paraplegia

112. 0.0!

John "Bluto" Blutarksy is the main protagonist of National Lampoon's Animal House. He is seven-year college student with a 0.0 grade average, Bluto is responsible for allocating fraternity identifiers to new members. After a period of service in the armed forces, Bluto served as a Senator, before becoming US President.

113. Barbie

Barbie's official birthday is March 9, 1959, the day she was unveiled to the toy industry during New York Toy Fair. Barbie first appeared in her iconic black-and-white striped swimsuit. Barbie was joined by Ken in 1961. The first Barbie doll was sold for $3.00.

114. Sissy Spacek

Sissy Spacek was the film's set dresser, assisting her then-boyfriend-now-husband Jack Fisk, the film's production designer. She later starred in De Palma's Carrie in 1976. A novelization of the film was written by Bjarne Rostaing.

115. The Walkman

The Walkman allowed people to take music with them wherever they went. It paved the way for the portable music devices that we still use today.

116. The Pink Ladies

We see Stephanie get off the school bus, and the rest of the Pink Ladies drive in, in their pink car! They all get out of the car and wonder where Stephanie is. Stephanie joins them, tells the Pink Ladies their going to be late, puts on her sunglasses and they all start doing a little dance!

117. Bell bottoms

The flared trouser supposedly has its origins in the US Navy, with American sailors being the first to adopt bell-bottomed trousers as early as 1817. They went for wide legs, due to the practicality of being able to roll up the legs when scrubbing the deck and easing removal when wet.

The pants symbolized the era, and you could see them everywhere, from the television screen to the streets around town.

118. Hans Solo

Smuggler. Scoundrel. Hero. Han Solo, captain of the Millennium Falcon, was one of the great leaders of the Rebel Alliance. He and his co-pilot Chewbacca came to believe in the cause of galactic freedom, joining Luke Skywalker and Princess Leia Organa in the fight against the Empire

119. Tom Selleck

George Lucas originally had his eyes on Tom Selleck before considering Ford to play Indiana Jones. But three weeks before filming began, Magnum, P.I.'s schedule forced the actor to drop out.

120. Gilligan's Island

The 98th and final episode of *Gilligan's Island* was broadcast on April 17, 1967. Though never a critical favorite, the show was still a solid rating hit and the cast and crew had every expectation of returning in the fall for the fourth season. But at the last minute, CBS needed to find some room on the schedule for *Gunsmoke*, the favorite show of Babe Paley, wife of network president William Paley. So, Gilligan got the ax and, at least as far as viewers know, the cast is still stranded somewhere in the Pacific.

121. Mack Lee Green - A Canadian former professional boxer who competed during the 1970s.

Carl Weathers wasn't the first choice for Rocky's Apollo Creed. Instead, there was a plan in place for a real-life boxer to play the character. A real-life boxer almost played Apollo Creed in Rocky. Instead, the iconic movie role went to Carl Weathers.

122. The Beatles

The band liked the idea of using the name of an insect as a band name, and they were fans of Buddy Holly and the Crickets. Because John Lennon loved puns, he altered the spelling of "Beetles" to "Beatles".

123. Donna Summer

How did she get her name? She was just a few weeks away from graduating from Jeremiah E. Burke High School in the Boston area when she auditioned for a production of "Hair" taking place in Germany. When word came that she'd been cast, the singer dropped out of high school and headed for Munich. She'd stick around Germany after "Hair" finished its run and strike up a romance with actor Helmuth Sommer. The couple later married, and the singer began going by the name Donna Sommer.

During the release of her first single, there was reportedly a printing mistake on the label, exchanging an "o" with a "u," and the result was Donna Summer. The name stuck.

124. Lava lamps

The lamp was invented by Edward Craven Walker, a British accountant. He was passing the time in a pub when he noticed a homemade egg timer crafted from a cocktail shaker filled with alien-looking liquids bubbling on a stove top. Determined to perfect the design, and to install a light bulb as the heat source, he settled on a bottle used for Orange Squash. The lamp paired two mutually insoluble liquids: one water-based, the other wax-based.

125. The Godfather

Actor Richard Castellano improvised that line after director Francis Ford Coppola added a line in an earlier scene in which Clemenza's wife says, "Don't forget the cannoli!"

126. Addis Ababa

Lex Luthor enters the Metropolis Museum of Natural History and steals the Addis Ababa L9 Pallasite Meteorite, which was discovered at the Kebe Mine in Addis Ababa, Ethiopia. It is described in the exhibit display as "sodium lithium boron silicate hydroxide with fluorine". According to the exhibit display, the meteorite was discovered in 1978 - the year that Superman: The Movie was released.

127. Hackensack.

When Superman is nearly killed after being given a huge pendant of green Kryptonite and left to drown, Luthor boasts of his plan to destroy California with the US Navy nuclear warhead Miss Teschmacher reprogrammed. He is sending a second missle to Hackensack, New Jersey, where Miss Teschmacher's mother lives. Miss Teschmacher expresses concern that her mother lives in Hackensack, to which Luthor callously remarks "Not for much longer" and leaves.

128. Atari 2600

The Atari 2600 was released in 1977. The games that you could play on the Atari 2600 included 'Street Racer' and 'Pac-Man' that are still loved today.

129. Stretch Armstrong

Stretch Armstrong was a toy filled with corn syrup. The doll was a wrestler-type figure that could be stretched from its original size.

130. Space Invaders

It was the first game to save and achieve high scores. Designer Nishikado drew inspiration from North American target shooting games like Breakout (1976) and the movie Star Wars (1977). Space Invaders is considered one of the most influential video games of all time. It helped expand the video game industry from a novelty to a global industry and ushered in the golden age of arcade video games.

131. Elvis Presley

Elvis Aaron Presley was born on January 8, 1935, in Tupelo, Mississippi, to Vernon Elvis and Gladys Love Presley in a two-room shotgun house that his father built for the occasion. Elvis's identical twin brother, Jesse Garon Presley, was delivered 35 minutes before him, stillborn.

132. The Twilight Zone

133. She saw blood

The girls were clearly thinking that Sandy was not as cool as them, having never smoked or really drank before. Frenchy offered to pierce her ears and insisted when Sandy was reluctant. They went into the bathroom, where a scream was heard. Frenchy then came out saying that Sandy got sick after seeing the blood. While Sandy was still in the bathroom, Rizzo and the girls sang "Look at Me, I'm Sandra Dee", poking fun at Sandy.

134. HBO (Home Box Office)

This venture led to the creation of a national satellite distribution system that used a newly approved domestic satellite transmission.

HBO subscribers paid an extra fee from the beginning. He local cable operators charged $6 for the HBO television channel. The company received $3.50 of them.

HBO was available from 3 p.m. until midnight for almost ten years. In 1981, however, the company started broadcasting 24/7 in order to compete with Showtime.

135. S.S. Minnow

Show creator Sherwood Schwartz named it thusly as an insult to then Chairman of the FCC (Federal Communications Commission). Mr. Minow, with one n. He did it because Mr. Minow had given a speech decrying television as a "vast wasteland" and how t.v. needed to improve its' standards.

136. Fats

Fats is the main antagonist in the 1978 psychological horror film Magic.
He is a ventriloquist dummy voiced by Corky Withers himself and portrayed by the actor Anthony Hopkins, who also played Hannibal Lecter in Silence of the Lambs and Ted Crawford in Fracture.

137. Beverly Johnson

The first African American to grace the cover of Vogue was Beverly Johnson. She has also been in a few movies and television shows throughout her career.

138. Platforms

The history of the platform begins around 600 BCE; the Greeks used them in plays, to increase the height of characters. High-status women also wore them. During the Middle Ages, the Venetians' platforms were called Chopines, while much of the rest of Europe's platforms were called Pattens.

Their modern popularization is credited to Italian shoe designer Salvatore Ferragamo. His rainbow sole hit the market in the 1930s, and it's been part of pop culture ever since. These platform sandals were made for Judy Garland in tribute to her performance of 'Over the Rainbow' in the Wizard of Oz.

139. Feathered Hair

The hair was layered and brushed outwards. Many celebrities sported this look at the time. Over the years, a lot of the credit has gone to celebrity hairstylist Allan Edwards. He claims to have given Fawcett her feathers way back in 1974, two years before she reached a national audience on the silver screen

140 Princess Leia

141. Pong

The engineer and developer that Atari had hired to create their video game had zero experience with video games. Allan Alcorn was hired initially to develop a driving video game, but since he had no prior experience developing games, Atari's co-founder Nolan Bushnell had Alcorn work on some practice code first to improve his skills. That practice project became the Pong game we know today.

142. Garfield

Garfield, the star, was based on the cats Davis grew up around; he took his name and personality from Davis' grandfather, James A. Garfield Davis, whom he described as "a large, cantankerous man." The name Jon Arbuckle came from a 1950s coffee commercial. Jon's roommate Lyman, added to give Jon someone to talk with, carried on the name of an earlier Gnorm Gnat character. The final character was Lyman's dog Spot, who was renamed Odie to avoid confusion with a dog also named Spot in the comic strip Boner's Ark.

143. Nostromo

Nostromo in Italian means boatswain, the officer in charge of the crew on a ship. The name conjures up a sense of responsibility based on that fact alone. In the novel, the character makes a name for himself as being reliable.

144. Nadia Comaneci

Initially, this decision led to a confusion of the public as the board flashed up '1.00' instead, the scoreboard having only three digits to display scores such as 9.50, or 9.85.

As no-one had ever achieved a perfect score in gymnastics until Nadia Comaneci at the 1976 Summer Olympics, she earned the nickname: the 'goddess from Montréal'. Over the course of her the Olympic careers, Comaneci would earn six additional 10s.

145. James Taylor

Drag racing east from Los Angeles in a souped-up '55 Chevy are the wayward Driver and Mechanic (singer-songwriter James Taylor and the Beach Boys' Dennis Wilson, in their only acting roles), accompanied by a tagalong Girl (Laurie Bird).

146. Fred

The Bassett Hound dog for Snowman's pet, was personally picked by Burt Reynolds, chiefly because it refused to obey commands.

147. MTV

At 12:01 a.m., on Saturday, August 1, 1981, Music Television (MTV) was launched with these words: "Ladies and gentlemen, rock and roll." In the 1980s, MTV was a pop culture juggernaut, with its VJs (video jockeys), music videos with style-conscious musical artists and the Video Music Awards (VMAs).

148. For Your Eyes Only (1981) and License to Kill (1989)

149. Erika Eleniak

Everyone remembers the science class scene in which Elliott (Henry Thomas) sets the frogs free and kisses his pretty blonde classmate (Erika Eleniak) in a cute recreation of John Wayne and Maureen O'Hara's big smooch from The Quiet Man.

150. EPCOT

On October 1, 1982, the Experimental Community of Tomorrow opened at Disney World. Walt Disney had envisioned EPCOT as an experimental planned urban community. Now it's a park with two parts: Future World, with cutting-edge pavilions like Spaceship Earth; and World Showcase, with pavilions showcasing 11 different countries.

151. What was the license number on the Ghostbusters' car?

152. Transforming the world of music and data storage, Sony was the first to sell this new digital music player in 1982.

153. In "Back to The Future" Christopher Lloyd hilariously portrays Dr. Emmett Brown, who invents time travel. What fuel does his time travel machine use?

154. What song recorded by Olivia Newton-John spent the most weeks at no.1 and became the most successful song on the Billboard in the 1980s?

155. In 1983, the world of communications was forever changed. Which big blocky device with a large antenna was first sold?

156. What does Ally Sheedy use to decorate her picture in the Breakfast Club?

157. One of the best-selling albums of the decades was Born in the U.S.A; who was this by?

158. In 'Dirty Dancing' what was Baby's real name?

159. What is the name of the Freelings' dog in "Poltergeist"?

160. What is the name of Sarah's brother that she is trying to save in "The Labyrinth"?

161. Two of the biggest computer companies were created in 1975 and 1976, by Bill and Steve respectively.

162. Which TV comedy series created by Jim Henson featuring a cast of puppet characters premiered on September 5, 1976?

163. For 39 years, Babe Ruth stood alone as baseball's all-time home run king. Then, on April 8, 1974, Ruth passed the torch to a new record holder. Who was he?

164. Which popular arcade game was based on the idea of "eating". The main character came about when the creator removed a slice from a pizza.

165. Name the 1980 British-American biographical drama film about Joseph Merrick (John Merrick in the film), a severely deformed man in late 19th-century London.

166. What is the name of a 1981 video game series featuring the adventures of a gorilla?

167. In the 1984 movie "Splash", the pretty blonde mermaid chooses which street name to be her own?

168. Which was the must-have watch of the '80s?

169. What is the name of the video game of two Italian twin brother plumbers who exterminate creatures emerging from the sewers by knocking them upside-down and kicking them away?

170. What is the name of Marty's band that tries out for the dance in Back to the Future?

171. Which famous video game, created by a Russian programmer, got its name from a combination of "tetra" (the Greek word meaning "four") and "tennis" (his favorite sport)?

172. What album released in 1982 has become the world's best-selling album? Tip: It is a little scary.

173. In the movie "Better Off Dead", what was the name of Lane's younger brother?

174. How many gigawatts of electricity did Doc Brown need to generate to power the DeLorean in Back to the Future?

175. What were the Ghostbusters' names?

176. In 1982, which computer was released as a home computer with several uses, and it would go on to be the highest-selling single computer model ever? Tip: Known also as the C64?

177. Cartoonist Hank Ketcham was pursuing a career in cartooning in 1950 when his first wife, Alice, once interrupted him to share the news that their four-year-old son had just demolished his bedroom by playing with the fecal matter found in his underpants declaring him a "menace". This inspired which cartoon?

178. What was the make and model of the villain in "The Terminator" 1984?

179. Which singer played the central character of the 1985 movie Desperately Seeking Susan?

180. What is the name of the main female character in 'The Terminator'?

181. Which colorful female character in a cartoon was an orphan and her real name was Wisp? Tip: Her nemesis was called Murky and owned a Color Belt.

182. What brand and color of underwear is Marty wearing in Back to the Future?

183. Which movie from 1983 influenced fashion with leggings, leg warmers and oversized sweatshirts? What a feeling!

184. What is the "Brat Pack"?

185. Which country won 83 gold medals and topped the 1984 Olympics medal table?

186. In The Karate Kid, what was Mr. Miyagi's yellow car?

187. What is it that first makes E.T.'s heart light go on?

188. What is the name of the candy that Eliot gives to E.T.?

189. Which sitcom depicted an alien on the planet Melmac?

190. Who won the first Rugby World Cup in 1987?

191. What is the name of the fictional place "where everybody knows your name"?

192. Name the 1988 American fantasy horror comedy film directed by **Tim Burton** starring **Michael Keaton** as the titular character. The plot revolves around a recently deceased couple who, as ghosts haunting their former home, contact an obnoxious and devious "bio-exorcist" from the Netherworld, to scare away the house's new inhabitants.

193. Three widows and a divorcée decided to live together in Miami. What's the name of this show? Fun fact: Eagle-eyed fans have noticed over the years that although there were four women living in the Miami house, there were always only three chairs around that famous kitchen table.

194. What does Allison Reynolds played by Ally Sheedy say she likes to drink in the Breakfast Club?

195. This character's favorite weapon was his whip, and his catch phrase was "We Do Not Follow Maps to Buried Treasure, And X Never, Ever Marks the Spot." Who is he?

196. Which basketball great was the NBA Rookie of the Year in 1985? Tip: He starred in a movie with Bugs Bunny.

197. Which hockey player is known as "The Great One"?

198. Which professional football team came out with a dance called "The Super Bowl Shuffle"?

199. In Beverly Hills Cop, how does Axel Foley escape the police car that is sent to follow him?

200. What kind of car does Nick Nolte's character in 48 hours?

ENTERTAINMENT & POP CULTURE

151. ECTO-1

The Ectomobile, or Ecto-1 is a 1959 Cadillac Miller-Meteor Sentinel limo-style endloader combination car (ambulance conversion) used in the 1984 film Ghostbusters and other Ghostbusters fiction. The original vehicle design was the creation of Steven Dane, credited as a Hardware Consultant in the credits.

152. The compact disc player.

Initially only in Japan, called the CDP-101. And they weren't cheap either - the player cost around $730 dollars.

153. Plutonium

He gets it from a group of Libyan terrorists (they wanted him to make a nuclear bomb).

154. Physical

It was released as the album's lead single on 28 September 1981. The song was written by Steve Kipner and Terry Shaddick, who had originally intended to offer it to Rod Stewart. The song had also been offered to Tina Turner by her manager Roger Davies, but when Turner declined, Davies gave the song to Newton-John, another of his clients.

It is the most successful single of Newton-John's career and became her fifth (and last) number-one single on the US Billboard Hot 100.

155. The first mobile phone

Cell phones are such a part of our lives now, especially as smartphones. But before the advent of the iPhone, there was the DynaTAC 8000x, the first commercially available mobile phone, costing $3,995 at the time. That big, blocky white phone with its large antenna was an iconic symbol of status, but that was mainly in the '90s.

156. Dandruf

Sheedy's most popular role to this day is still Allison, the "basket case" in "The Breakfast Club." In one memorable scene, her oddball character uses her own dandruff to decorate her drawing as "snow."

157. Bruce Springsteen

Born in the U.S.A. became his most commercially successful album and one of the highest-selling records ever, having sold 30 million copies by 2012. It has also been cited by critics as one of the greatest albums of all time. The album received a nomination for Album of the Year at the 1985 Grammy Awards.

158. Frances Houseman

Spending the summer at a Catskills resort with her family, Frances "Baby" Houseman falls in love with the camp's dance instructor, Johnny Castle.

159. E.Buzz

Buzz is actually the first member of the Freeling family that we meet. The film opens with the TV turning to static as the broadcast ends. Dad Steven (Craig T. Nelson) is snoozing in an armchair in front of the TV while the dog cleans up whatever was left on the plate next to Steven's chair.

160. Toby

Sixteen-year-old Sarah is given thirteen hours to solve a labyrinth and rescue her baby brother Toby when her wish for him to be taken away is granted by the Goblin King Jareth.

161. Microsoft was created on April 4, 1975, by Bill Gates and Apple on April 1, 1976, by Steve Jobs.

Inspired by the January cover of Popular Electronics magazine, friends Bill Gates and Paul Allen started Microsoft, sometimes Micro-Soft, for microprocessors and software, to develop software for the Altair 8800, an early personal computer.

Jobs became bent on starting a company of his own to build computers for individuals, and he convinced Wozniak to start it with him. They sold some of their prized belongings – for Jobs, a Volkswagen minibus, and for Wozniak, a programmable HP calculator – to raise $1300 to launch the enterprise.

162. The Muppet Show ran from 1976 to 1981.

It featured the Muppets, a cast of puppet characters that included Kermit the Frog, Miss Piggy, Fozzie Bear, and Gonzo, as they prepared for their weekly vaudeville show.

Fun fact. The original incarnation of Kermit the Frog was dubbed Kermit the Thing. Henson, its creator, confirmed that Kermit was actually made out of his mother's old coat and that "I didn't call him a frog … all the characters in those days were abstract because that was part of the principle that I was working under, that you wanted abstract things."

163. Hank Aaron

Aaron had been working toward this moment for 20 years. His first home run came in his rookie season, on April 23, 1954, with the Milwaukee Braves.

After his momentous home run, Aaron hit 40 more dingers before retiring in 1976, with 755 career homers and his Hall of Fame candidacy sealed many times over.

164. Pac Man

In 1980 the Japanese arcade game manufacturer Namco Limited introduced the world to Pac-Man. The lead designer was Iwatani Tohru, who intended to create a game that did not emphasize violence.

The original Japanese name was Puckman, which evolved from the Japanese word paku, meaning "chomp." Given the closeness to a certain explicit four-letter English word, a lot of arcade operators at the time were worried that vandals would alter the letter P. Eventually, "Pac" was suggested as an alternate name.

165. The Elephant Man

The Elephant Man was a critical and commercial success with eight **Academy Award** nominations.

Joseph Carey Merrick (5 August 1862 – 11 April 1890), often erroneously called John Merrick, was an English man born in **Leicester** who began to develop abnormally before the age of five. His mother died when he was eleven and his father soon remarried. Rejected by his father and stepmother, he left home and went to live with his uncle Charles Merrick.

In 1884, he contacted a showman named **Sam Torr** and proposed that Torr should exhibit him. Torr arranged for a group of men to manage Merrick, whom they named "the Elephant Man".

Although the official cause of his death was **asphyxia**, Treves, who performed the **postmortem**, said Merrick had died of a dislocated neck.

166. Donkey Kong

The first game was the 1981 arcade game Donkey Kong, featuring the eponymous character as the main antagonist in an industrial construction setting and the debut of both the Donkey Kong and **Mario** characters. The game was a massive success and was followed by two sequels released in 1982 and 1983.

167. Madison

The mermaid in "Splash" sees a sign marking Madison Avenue, and she immediately decides that her name will be Madison.

168. Swatch

Swiss watchmaker Swatch came on the scene in the U.S. in 1983, with dazzling colors and styles, plastic straps and Swiss movement. Swatch meant "second watch," a watch for more casual wear, and it's arguably the watch of the 1980s.

169. Mario Bros

Mario is a character created by Japanese video game designer Shigeru Miyamoto. Mario first appeared as the player character of Donkey Kong (1981), a platform game. Miyamoto wanted to use Popeye as the protagonist, but when he could not achieve the licensing rights, he created Mario instead.

Depicted as a short, pudgy Italian plumber who resides in the Mushroom Kingdom, his adventures generally center on rescuing Princess Peach from the Koopa villain Bowser. Mario has access to a variety of power-ups that give him different abilities. Mario's fraternal twin brother is Luigi.

170. The Pinheads

The Pinheads was a band, consisting of Marty McFly, Paul, Lee, and Bobby.

171. Tetris

Tetris is a puzzle video game created by Soviet software engineer Alexey Pajitnov in 1984. Pajitnov was inspired by a puzzle game called "pentominoes," in which different wooden shapes made of five equal squares are assembled in a box.

The Tetris theme song is an instrumental arrangement of a Russian folk tune called "Korobeiniki." The song is so famous that it is now a registered sound mark in the U.S. and other countries.

172. "Thriller" by Michael Jackson

"Thriller" was released on November 30, 1982, and was part of the zeitgeist of 1980s music, with Jackson's music videos on heavy rotation on MTV. "Thriller" won eight Grammys in 1984, including the Album of the Year. To date, Thriller has sold 66 million copies.

173. Badger

Lane lives in a suburban development with his mother, Jenny, a ditzy housewife who routinely concocts creepy (and creeping) family meals; his genius little brother, Badger, who never speaks but at the age of "almost 8" can build powerful lasers.

174. 1.21 gigawatts!!

175. Peter Venkman (Bill Murray), Egon Spengler (Harold Ramis), Ray Stantz (Dan Ackroyd), and Winston Zedmore (Ernie Hudson)

176. Commodore 64

It has been listed in the Guinness Book of World Records as one of the best-selling single computer models of all time.

The C64 dominated the low-end computer market for most of the 1980s. For a substantial period (1983–1986), the C64 had between 30% and 40% share of the US market and two million units sold per year, outselling the IBM PC compatibles, Apple Inc. computers, and the Atari 8-bit family of computers.

177. Dennis the Menace.

Ketcham's son may have outgrown his bedroom-destroying habits, but a series of misfortunes led to a life far more chaotic than his cartoon counterpart. Expelled from boarding school, Dennis Ketcham served in Vietnam and suffered from post-traumatic stress disorder. He and his father reportedly had little contact prior to the elder Ketcham's death in 2001.

The cartoonist once commented he had some regrets about naming his creation after Dennis, saying it "confused" his son. Talking with *People* in 1993, Dennis said he wished his father "could have used something other than my childhood for his ideas."

178. T-800 Cyberdyne Systems Model 101

A Cyberdyne Systems Model 101 Terminator with living tissue over a metal endoskeleton, played by Schwarzenegger, is the main antagonist of The Terminator, the original Terminator film. Another Model 101, having been reprogrammed by the human resistance in the future, is the protagonist of Terminator 2: Judgment Day.

179. Madonna

The filmmakers considered Diane Keaton and Goldie Hawn to play Susan and Roberta, respectively. The characters were of a different generation. Susan was more of a hippie traveler, Diane Keaton in an embroidered shirt. The downtown Susan story, pyramid jacket, and Nefertiti earrings came later.

However, when the producers decided to reimagine Susan as a New Wave/Punk figure, they first considered Melanie Griffith, Jennifer Jason Leigh, Ellen Barkin, and Kelly McGillis.

180. Sarah

Sarah is destined to give birth to a man named John Connor who will grow up lead the human resistance against The Machines. The future of the human race relies on her.

181. Rainbow Brite

Her name only changed to Rainbow Brite in the cartoon series' second episode after she defeated the Dark One and became the keeper of the Color Belt.

182. Purple Calvin Klein briefs

Basic outfit. During most of his adventures, except when he changed clothes in 1955 and 1885, Marty wore Guess blue jeans with black 3/4" suspenders, a red t-shirt, lavender ("purple") Calvin Klein underpants, and white Nike Bruin shoes with red swoosh and back tab (no word Nike on them until he visited 1885) with gray socks (changed to white socks when he visited 2015).

183. Flashdance

Jennifer Beals' portrayal of a young welder trying to make it as a professional dancer in "Flashdance" was an instant classic, despite negative reviews from critics. After that movie debuted, leg warmers and leggings became a new fashion trend.

184. The term "Brat Pack", a play on the Rat Pack from the 1950s and 1960s, was first popularized in a 1985 New York magazine cover story, which described a group of highly successful film stars in their early twenties. It was a group of young actors who frequently appeared together in teen-oriented coming-of-age films in the 1980s.

The "core" members are considered to be Emilio Estevez, Anthony Michael Hall, Rob Lowe, Andrew McCarthy, Demi Moore, Judd Nelson, Molly Ringwald, Andrew McCarthy, and Ally Sheedy.

185. USA

The 1984 Summer Olympics were held in Los Angeles, California, United States, from July 28 to August 12. Athletes from host nation United States won the most medals overall with 174 and the most gold medals with 83.

It marked the first time the United States led the medal count in both gold and overall medals since 1968.Many writers and sports commentators noted that the absence of the Soviet Union and various other Eastern Bloc nations stemming from a boycott contributed to the highly skewed medal results favoring the United States.

186. Yellow 1947 Ford Super Deluxe Convertible

The Yellow Car used in the famous "Wax On-Wax Off" Scene, which was given to Daniel by Miyagi in the film, was actually given to actor Ralph Macchio as a gift from the film's producer. He stills owns the car today.

187. He hears an owl hoot.

All their heart lights go on when the owl makes noise.

188. Reese's Pieces

When Elliot tries to lure his newfound friend out into the backyard, he uses some candy that he has on hand, the Hersey's candy, Reese's Pieces. He places pieces of the brown, orange, and yellow chocolate for E.T. to munch on.

This wouldn't be the only food that E.T. enjoys throughout the movie. When Elliot goes to school, E.T. explores the house (and the fridge) on his own and ends up drinking quite a few beers. This doesn't turn out well for the duo, but in the end, their friendship keeps them connected.

189. ALF

ALF is an alien from the planet Melmac who has arrived on planet Earth, and lands in the Tanner family's garage. On Melmac, ALF was a member of the planet's Orbit Guard. He was given the nickname "ALF", by Willie Tanner in the pilot episode, an acronym short for Alien Life Form.

190. New Zealand

The first tournament took place in May and June 1987, with games played in both New Zealand and Australia. The final was held at Eden Park, Auckland, on 20 June, with the home team beating France 29–9 to become the inaugural holders of the Webb Ellis Cup.

191. Cheers

"Cheers" was a popular sitcom about bar regulars in a bar modeled after a real bar in Boston. "Cheers" made its debut in 1982 but was almost canceled in its first season when it ranked near the bottom of the Nielsen ratings. It's arguably one of the most popular and critically acclaimed TV series to date.

192. Beetlejuice

Beetlejuice opened theatrically in the United States on March 30, 1988, earning US$8,030,897 in its opening weekend. The film eventually grossed US$73,707,461 in North America. Beetlejuice was a financial success, recouping its US$15 million budget, and was the 10th-highest grossing film of 1988

193. The Golden Girls

We all know their names: Dorothy, Sophia, Rose and Blanche. "The Golden Girls" debuted in 1985 and spun off three shows: "Golden Palace," "Empty Nest" and "Nurses." "Golden Girls" won many awards and critical acclaim, and the show still influences popular culture today.

194. Vodka

She spends the first half of the movie in almost complete silence. However, when she does start talking, almost everything she says needs to be taken with a pinch of salt, given her predilection for making stuff up.

This scene takes place over thirty minutes into the movie, and Allison hasn't spoken up until this point (apart from a "Ha!"). When Andrew asks her what she drinks, she breaks her silence and says, "Vodka."

195. Indiana Jones

The character was originally named Indiana Smith, after an Alaskan Malamute called Indiana that Lucas owned in the 1970s and on which he based the Star Wars character Chewbacca. Spielberg disliked the name Smith, and Lucas casually suggested Jones as an alternative.

196. Michael Jordan

Michael Jordan's NBA debut with the Chicago Bulls was as the number-three draft pick. In 1986, after overcoming a broken foot earlier in the season, he set the still-standing record of 63 points in a playoff game. His six NBA Championship rings came in the '90s, but Jordan was already on his way to being one of the greatest basketball players of all time.

197. Wayne Gretzky

You can't talk about the National Hockey League, or hockey in general, and not mention Wayne Gretzky. He utterly dominated the NHL, with records involving scoring goals, assists and MVP awards. During the '80s he was with the Edmonton Oilers, until he was traded to the Los Angeles Kings in 1988.

198. Chicago Bears

The 1985 Chicago Bears, who won Super Bowl XX against the New England Patriots, have been called one of the greatest football teams of all time. "Da Bears" were led by head coach Mike Ditka, along with memorable players like running back Walter "Sweetness" Payton and defensive lineman William "Refrigerator" Perry. "The Super Bowl Shuffle" was a rap song the team recorded, which made it to #41 on Billboard's Hot 100.

199. He puts a banana in its tailpipe.

The banana in the tail pipe was a last second food choice. In the script, Axel stuffs potatoes he stole from the hotel kitchen into the tail pipe of Rosewood and Taggart's car. Due to time constraints, no scene from the kitchen could be shot. Because the hotel lobby was already a location for a few scenes, the script was re-written, so Axel takes bananas, with Damon Wayans' approval, from a buffet in the lobby.

200. The make and model of Jack Cates (Nick Nolte)'s car is a sky blue 1964 Cadillac DeVille convertible.

The nickname Hammond calls the car is a "piece of shit sky-blue Cadillac". Hammond's (Eddie Murphy) car was said to be a Porsche, meaning a Porsche 356 Speedster, but the vehicle is actually an Intermeccanica 356 A Speedster replica built by CMC (Classic Motor Carriage).

201. What famous director makes a cameo appearance in the Blues Brothers?

202. In the 1983 movie "National Lampoon's Vacation," where were the Griswolds headed on their cross country trip?

203. In the movie "Stand by Me", what did Gordie, Chris, Vern and Teddy set out to find?

204. Which 1987 Whitney Houston single became her first US platinum-selling single?

205. Which team was Magic Johnson part of in the '80s?

206. In the movie "Tootsie" what was the name of the woman who was played by cross-dressing Dustin Hoffmann?

207. Rick Deckard is a special agent in the Los Angeles police department employed to hunt down and "retire" replicants. What is his profession referred to as? Tip: It is also the name of this futuristic movie directed by Ridley Scott.

208. What is the line in Labyrinth that Sarah can never remember?

209. What was the name of the prison mouse in the movie 'The Green Mile'?

210. Name the charity song written in 1984 by Bob Geldof and Midge Ure to raise money for the 1983–1985 famine in Ethiopia. Tip: It was first recorded by Band Aid.

211. Which female tennis player achieved the "Golden Slam" in 1988?

212. Homer, Bart, Lisa, and Maggie first made their appearance in 1987 in a US animated sitcom created by Matt Groening for Fox. What is the name of this sitcom?

213. Numerous expeditions had tried to locate this famous shipwreck using sonar to map the seabed but had been unsuccessful. In 1985, the wreck was finally found. Name the ship.

201. Steven Spielberg.

Look for him at the end of the film in the office of the county assessor. A number of non-musicians managed to make their way into the film as well including Frank Oz and Twiggy.

202. WalleyWorld

203. The body of a boy who had been hit by a train.

Gordie, Chris, and Teddy learn from Vern that Ray Brower's dead body has been found, apparently killed after being struck by a train. Ray Brower was a young boy whose death and subsequent police search created a big news story in Castle Rock.

The film ends shortly after the boys find the body. After their run-in with Ace, where Gordie turns a gun on the cruel thug, they head home. As they reach their hometown of Castle Rock (the location of many a Stephen King story), they say their goodbyes to one another.

204. I Wanna Dance with Somebody

It received mixed reviews from music critics, who praised Houston's vocal performance but critiqued its musical arrangement comparing it to Houston's own "How Will I Know" and Cyndi Lauper's "Girls Just Want to Have Fun." Despite the mixed critical response, the song became a worldwide success, topping the charts in eighteen countries including Australia, Italy, Germany and the UK. In the US,

205. Los Angeles Lakers

In 1974 he earned the nickname "Magic" after a game his sophomore year of high school, in which he scores 36 points, 18 rebounds and 16 assists. Lansing State Journal sportswriter Fred Stabley Jr. is the first to call him Magic.

He helped the Lakers win five NBA championships: 1980, 1982, 1985, 1987 and 1988.

206. Dorothy Michaels

Being the die-hard method actor that he is, Hoffman would take such an approach in real life to ensure his female impersonation was convincing. For one, the actor went to his daughter's parents' evening at school as "Aunt Dorothy," and reportedly the teachers never suspected it was Hoffman.

207. Blade Runner

Police units, called "blade runners", have the job of destroying - or in their parlance "retiring" - any replicant that makes its way back to or created on Earth.
The replicants need to be killed because they are a threat to humanity. They are designed to be perfect copies of humans, but they have a limited lifespan of just four years. This means that they could eventually outnumber humans and take over the world.

208. You have no power over me!

The Labyrinth is only known through the lines Sarah recites from it in the film. The most important speech in the play is the one Sarah says aloud at the start of the film, and later must recite at the end of the film to defeat Jareth.

Through dangers untold and hardships unnumbered,
I have fought my way here
To the castle beyond the Goblin City,
To take back the child that you have stolen,
For my will is as strong as yours,
And my kingdom is as great.
<u>You have no power over me.</u>

209. Mr. Jingles.

The mouse was called Mr. Jingles in The Green Mile, less frequently, Steamboat Willie. When death row inmate Eduard Delecroix finds the mouse in the prison, he names it Mr. Jingles and keeps it as a pet and companion in his cell.

210. Do They Know It's Christmas?

"Do They Know It's Christmas?" was rerecorded and rereleased in 1989, 2004 and 2014. The 1989 and 2004 versions also raised funds for famine relief, while the 2014 version raised funds for the Ebola crisis in West Africa. All three reached number one in the UK, and the 1989 and 2004 versions became Christmas number ones. The 2004 version sold 1.8 million copies.

211. Steffi Graf

On October 1, 1988, Steffi Graf defeated Gabriela Sabatini in the singles final of the Olympic tournament in Seoul (6-3, 6-3). Three weeks after completing the calendar Grand Slam, the German had just added a gold medal to make her season even greater. This feat would remain as a "Golden Slam", an expression that was specifically invented to define this unique achievement and would make Graf's 1988 season the greatest ever played in tennis.

212. The Simpsons

Why are they yellow?

When Matt Groening was creating The Simpsons, he wanted the family to stand out, so he decided to make the characters a weird color. "An animator came up with the Simpsons' yellow and as soon as she showed it to me I said: 'This is the answer!' " Groening once told the BBC.

213. The Titanic

Almost immediately after Titanic sank on 15 April 1912, proposals were advanced to salvage her from her resting place in the North Atlantic Ocean, despite her exact location and condition being unknown. The families of several wealthy victims of the disaster, the Guggenheims, Astors, and Wideners, formed a consortium and contracted the Merritt and Chapman Derrick and Wrecking Company to raise Titanic.

The project was soon abandoned as impractical as the divers could not even reach a significant fraction of the necessary depth, where the pressure is over 6,000 pounds per square inch (40 megapascals). The lack of submarine technology at the time as well as the outbreak of World War I also put off such a project

GENERAL KNOWLEDGE

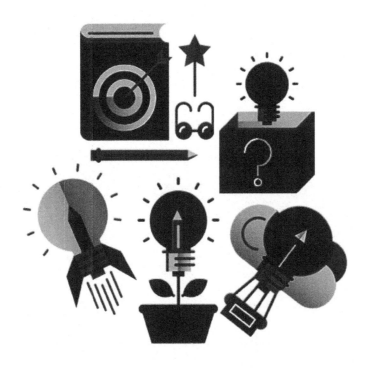

QUESTIONS 1 - 50
GENERAL KNOWLEDGE

1. How long is the Golden Gate bridge?

2. How many stars are in our solar system?

3. When did World War I begin?

4. How many planets are in our solar system? Name the in order.

5. Who is the writer of Harry Potter?

6. Who was the first woman pilot?

7. Who is the inventor of the basketball hoop?

8. What is Han Solo's ship called in Star Wars?

9. What year did the Titanic sink?

10. Which city hosted the first Olympics?

11. What baseball team has won the most MLB championships?

12. What is the solar system's hottest planet?

13. What American football team went the entire 1972 season without any losses?

14. George Harrison was part of what popular musical group?

15. Where is the great barrier reef located and how long is it?

16. Who played "Jack" in the film, "Titanic?"

17. What country gifted the United States the Statue of Liberty?

18. How many bones are there in the adult human body? And how many are there in an infant's body?

19. How many sports are played in the Summer Olympic Games?

20. How many points was an American football touchdown worth in the year 1911?

21. Which portion of the plant is responsible for photosynthesis?

22. What is the only fruit to bear seeds on the outside?

23. What was ice cream once called?

24. Are peanuts a nut? True or false?

25. What plant family are cherries from?

26. Why do apples float in water?

27. How many weeks are in a year?

28. What sport did Abe Lincoln play before he was president?

29. Who was the first player to hit a home run in the All-Star game of 1933?

30. Why are clouds white?

31. What electric weather event can be five times hotter than the sun?

32. What year did tropical storms and hurricanes start earning names?

33. Name the only planet to spin clockwise?

34. How long are Neptune's days?

35. Which planet has the shortest days?

36. How long will the footprints on the moon be there?

37. What was the name of the first chimpanzee in space?

38. Where was the largest fossil spider found?

39. Where are more than 10% of a cat's bones located?

40. Where is a shrimp's heart?

41. What part of an Ostrich is larger than its brain?

42. What body part does a fox use to communicate?

43. What year did Wilt Chamberlain score 100 points in a single NBA game?

44. Why is Laika famous for?

45. How many seams are on an American baseball?

46. What are nails made of?

47. What never stops growing on your body?

48. What city in the United States has microclimates?

49. What is the largest ocean on Earth?

50. What are the 3 rarest blood types?

25. The rose family

Prunus, genus of more than 400 species of flowering shrubs and trees in the rose family (Rosaceae). The genus Prunus is native to northern temperate regions. It has a number of economically important members, including the cultivated almond, peach, plum, cherry, and apricot.

26. Because they're 1/4 air

Apples can float because 25% of their volume is air. If an item is denser than water it will sink, if it is less dense it will float. Apples are less dense than water, so they float!

27. 52 weeks

A year has 52 weeks plus 1 day. One calendar year has 365 days, which are divided into 7-day weeks. To know how many weeks there are in a year, you just divide the number of days there are in a year (365) by how many days there are in a week (7).

The result will be the average number of weeks there are in a year, which is approximately 52.143, or 52 weeks plus 1 day.

Every four years there is a leap year, which has 366 days. By the same calculations, we can understand that in leap years there are 52 weeks and 2 days.

28. Wrestling

He competed in wrestling matches for more than a decade of his youth and rarely lost. His abilities were formally recognized by the National Wrestling Hall of Fame, which inducted him as an "Outstanding American" in the sport in 1992.

29. Babe Ruth

In the bottom of the third, after a walk to Charlie Gehringer, Babe Ruth famously hit the first home run in All-Star Game history, putting the AL up 3–0.

30. Because they are reflecting sunlight above them.

Clouds are white because light from the Sun is white. As light passes through a cloud, it interacts with the water droplets, which are much bigger than the atmospheric particles that exist in the sky.

31. Lightning

Air is a very poor conductor of electricity and gets extremely hot when lightning passes through it. In fact, lightning can heat the air it passes through to 50,000 degrees Fahrenheit (5 times hotter than the surface of the sun).

32. 1953

Since 1953, Atlantic tropical storms had been named from lists originated by the National Hurricane Center. They are now maintained and updated through a strict procedure by an international committee of the World Meteorological Organization.

33. Venus

Unlike the other planets in our solar system, Venus spins clockwise on its axis. All other planets spin counter-clockwise on their axis and orbit the Sun in a counter-clockwise direction. It also means that if you could stand on the surface of Venus, the Sun would rise in the west and set in the east.

An explanation for the backward, or retrograde, rotation is not certain. A long-held theory is that Venus once rotated as the other planets do but was struck billions of years ago by a planet-size object. The impact and its aftermath caused the rotation to change directions or flipped the planetary axis.

34 16 hours long

A planet's day is the time it takes the planet to rotate or spin once on its axis. \ Neptune rotates faster than Earth so a day on Neptune is shorter than a day on Earth.

35. Jupiter

Jupiter has the shortest day of all the planets. A day on Jupiter lasts only nine hours and 55 minutes.

36. A million years (forever)

The first footprints on the Moon will be there for a million years. There is no wind to blow them away.

37. Ham, which stood for "Holloman Aero Medical"

On January 31, 1961, Ham became the first chimpanzee in space. On January 31, 1961, at Cape Canaveral, FL, 3 ½ year old Ham was propelled into space, strapped into a container called a "couch." Ham's flight lasted approximately 16 ½ minutes. He travelled at a speed of approximately 5800 mph, to a height of 157 miles above the earth. He experienced about 6 ½ minutes of weightlessness. Incredibly, despite the intense speed, g-forces, and weightlessness, Ham performed his tasks correctly.

When he was finally released from the "couch" however, his face bore an enormous grin. Although interpreted as a happy smile by many people, Ham's expression was one of extreme fear and anxiety.

38. China

Scientists have unearthed the largest spider fossil ever found. The spider, a new species called Nephila jurassica, stretches about two inches from end to end. It was found in a fossil-rich rock formation near Daohugou village in northeastern China

39. In its tail

A cat's tail contains almost 10 percent of their bones and serves as a counterweight to keep that graceful balance while they navigate a narrow space or makes sudden turns.

40. In its head

They have their hearts, along with other vital organs such as their stomach and ventral nerve cord, inside of their heads due to the safety this part of the body provides over the tail-end.

Their head and thorax are the thickest and hardest parts of the body. This section, known as the cephalic portion, is covered with a thick protective substance, known as an exoskeleton. This exoskeleton guards the shrimp's internal organs against harm, as damage to any of them could be fatal. Shrimp have evolved this way over time to help guarantee their survival.

41. Its eye

An ostrich's eye is bigger than its brain. Compared to other birds, ostriches aren't the smartest, but they have excellent eyesight. Their eyeballs measure two inches across and are about the size of a billiard ball.

42. They're tail

A fox uses its tail (or "brush") as a warm cover in cold weather and as a signal flag to communicate with other foxes. Foxes also signal each other by making scent posts, urinating on trees or rocks to announce their presence.

43. 1962

"The Big Dipper" dropped 100 points in 48 minutes of work as the Philadelphia Warriors defeated the New York Knicks on March 2, 1962.

44. Laika is the name of a dog launched into space by the Soviet Union (now Russia) in 1957.

She was not the first living creature in space, but she was the first to orbit the Earth. Officially, Laika was poisoned through her food after about a week to prevent a painful death when reentering the Earth's atmosphere.

45. 108 seams

In 1934 the MLB adopted a league-wide standard which has gone largely unchanged today: 108 double-stitches of waxed red thread.

46. Keratin

Keratin is a type of protein that forms the cells that make up the tissue in nails and other parts of your body.

Keratin forms the cells of your hair and skin, too. It also forms cells that are a key part of many glands and that line internal organs.

Nails start growing under your skin. As new cells grow, they push old ones through your skin. The part you can see consists of dead cells. That's why it doesn't hurt to cut your nails.

47. Your nose and ears

Our noses and ears are unique compared to the rest of our bodies because they're composed of soft tissue enveloped in cartilage. And it's this soft tissue that keeps growing throughout our entire lives. "When you look at someone when they're 80 vs. when they're 20, they'll have more cells in their ears and nose.

48. San Francisco

San Francisco is a city with microclimates and sub microclimates. Due to the city's varied topography and influence from the prevailing summer marine layer, weather conditions can vary by as much as 9 °F (5 °C) from block to block.

49. The Pacific Ocean

The Pacific Ocean is the largest and deepest of the world ocean basins. Covering approximately 63 million square miles and containing more than half of the free water on Earth, the Pacific is by far the largest of the world's ocean basins. All of the world's continents could fit into the Pacific basin.

50.

AB- (AB negative) blood type, which is seen in just 0.6 percent of people followed by.

B- (found in 1.5 percent of the United States population) and.
AB+ (present in just 3.4 percent of people in the United States).

GENERAL KNOWLEDGE

51. Who officially made Valentine's Day a holiday?

52. In what Italian city did Romeo and Juliet live?

53. What was the first company to put Santa Claus on a soda?

54. Where do Acai berries originate from?

55. How many cells does the human body contain?

56. How many different types of cells are in the human body?

57. What is the oldest known blood type?

58. Your blood is as salty as the ocean, true or false?

59. What is the tallest building in the world?

60. In what city is the White House located?

61. What is the largest continent on the planet?

62. What part of the world is the only place bees cannot be found?

63. What is the world's tallest mountain?

64. Name at least two animals that sleep standing up.

65. Humans have unique fingerprints and what else? Tip: The answer may be one body part and up to four (maybe even more).

66. What is the hardest rock on earth?

67. What percentage of Earth is covered in water?

68. Why are flamingos pink?

69. What is the full moon of spring referred to as?

70. What percentage of water is the human body?

71. What direction can kangaroos not walk?

72. Tiger's skin is striped like its fur, true or false?

73. How do frogs drink water?

74. How long does the average yawn last?

75. What is Thailand's capital city?

76. How many muscles are in the human body?

77. What is a group of frogs called?

78. What's a group of foxes called?

79. What fruit do humans share 50% of their DNA with?

80. What is the only bird that can fly backward?

81. Where did french fries originate from?

82. How many smells can the human nose smell?

83. What color blood does an octopus have?

84. Name the animal that has three hearts and nine brains.

85. What year was the first pizza delivery made?

86. What does the word "astronaut" mean in Greek?

87. What was the nationality of Marco Polo?

88. Where did hummingbirds get their name?

89. What is a group of jellyfish called?

90. What animal laughs when it's tickled?

91. What parts of our body contains traces of gold?

92. Who was the first president of the United States?

93. Who was the first person to win a Nobel Peace prize?

94. When was the first world cup played?

95. Why is July 4th a famous day in the U.S.?

96. What do you call a group of pigs?

97. What type of dog does the royal family famously own?

98. In a polo match, how many chukkers are there?

99. What is the temperature at which water boils?

100. What connects the muscles with the bones?

51. Henry VIII

King Henry VIII declared Valentine's Day an official holiday in 1537. The oldest handwritten Valentine was made in the 1400s and is held in the British Museum.

52. The Italian city of Verona

Although Shakespeare never visited Verona and his characters in Romeo & Juliet never existed, there is a 13th Century house in Verona where Juliet is said to have lived. It once belonged to the Capello family for many years.

53. Coca-Cola

Coca-Cola helped shape the image of Santa. So, Coca-Cola commissioned Michigan-born illustrator Haddon Sundblom to develop advertising images using Santa Claus, showing Santa himself, not a man dressed as Santa.

54. South America

The acai palm tree, native to tropical Central and South America, produces a deep purple fruit. The acai fruit has long been an important food source for indigenous peoples of the Amazon region.

55. 30 trillion cells

Scientists have come a long way in estimating the number of cells in the average human body. Most recent estimates put the number of cells at around 30 trillion. Written out, that's 30,000,000,000,000!

56. 200 different types

Here are just a few examples:
- red blood cells (erythrocytes)
- skin cells
- neurons (nerve cells)
- fat cells

Humans are multicellular, complex organisms. The cells inside our bodies are "specialized." This means that each type of cell performs a unique and special function. For this reason, each of the 200 different types of cells in the body has a different structure, size, shape, and function, and contains different organelles.

57. Type A

In molecular history, type A appears to be the 'oldest' blood type, in the sense that the mutations that gave rise to types O and B appear to stem from it. Geneticists call this the wild-type or ancestral allele.

58. True

Not only is blood mostly water, but the watery portion of blood, the plasma, has a concentration of salt and other ions that is remarkably similar to sea water.

59. Burj Khalifa

Known as the Burj Dubai prior to its inauguration in 2010, is a skyscraper in Dubai, United Arab Emirates. With a total height of 829.8 m (2,722 ft, or just over half a mile) and a roof height (excluding antenna but including a 223 m spire) of 828m (2,717 ft), the Burj Khalifa has been the tallest structure and building in the world since its topping out in 2009, supplanting Taipei 101, the previous holder of that status.

60. Washington, D.C.

The White House is located at 1600 Pennsylvania Avenue in Washington, D.C., the capital of the United States. The Washington Monument, the Capitol Building, the Jefferson Memorial, the Pentagon, and the Lincoln Memorial are also in the Washington, D.C. area.

61. Asia

Earth is covered by three-fourths ocean waters. The remaining land is mostly split into seven main divisions. These continents are Asia, Europe, North America, South America, Antarctica, Africa and Australia. Among the seven, Asia is the biggest continent by land size.

Asia stretches from the East Mediterranean Sea to the Western Pacific Ocean, with an area of approximately 45 million square kilometers, Guinness World Records report. The continent holds more than 40 countries, including China and India which are world's two most populous countries.

62. Antarctica

Antarctica is the only continent that's completely devoid of any bees. Of course, with temperatures reaching as low as minus 76 degrees Fahrenheit, not many living things can survive down there. In fact, most of the insects living in Antarctica are parasites, the kind that lives in the fur of sea animals or birds.

63. Everest

Mount Everest, located in Nepal and Tibet, is usually said to be the highest mountain on Earth. Reaching 29029 feet (8,848 meters) above mean sea level.

64. Horses, zebras, and elephants. Cows can too.

Horses, zebras and elephants sleep standing up. Cows can too, but mostly choose to lie down. Some birds also sleep standing up. Flamingos live on caustic salt flats, where there is no where they can sit down.

65. Tongue prints, iris of eyes, ears, and DNA

Move over fingerprints. From your ears to your toes, many of your body parts make you uniquely special. And all of them are being investigated as a way to identify you from others in a crowd.

It turns out the ridges, bumps and shape of your outer ear are so unique that it may soon be one of the best ways to identify you.

While your DNA does set the ultimate color and structure of each iris, the furrows, rifts and pits you see happen randomly during fetal development in the womb. It's called "chaotic morphogenesis," and is thought to occur when iris tissue tightens and folds as the fetus opens and shuts its developing eyes.

The bumps contain more than 10,000 taste buds, each one filled with microscopic hairs called microvilli. Microvilli function like tiny food critics, sensing if your meal is sweet or sour, salty or bitter, and sending reviews up to the brain.

Think of your DNA as four Legos that like to play in pairs along a spiral staircase called a double helix. Those pairs (A and T; C and G) form building blocks of code called genes that become the blueprint for your hair, eyes, body shape and everything else that makes you unique.

Your voice, the way you walk, and even teeth are also unique to you.

66. Diamond

Diamond is the hardest known mineral. It is a high-symmetry allotrope of carbon (C). It has a Mohs "scratch" hardness of 10, which makes it the hardest mineral.

The Mohs scale of mineral hardness is a qualitative ordinal scale, from 1 to 10, characterizing scratch resistance of various minerals through the ability of harder material to scratch softer material.

67. 70%

About 71% of the Earth's surface is water-covered, and the oceans hold about 96.5 percent of all Earth's water. Water also exists in the air as water vapor, in rivers and lakes, in icecaps and glaciers, in the ground as soil moisture and in aquifers, and even in you and your dog.

68. They're not really. Well, not at birth, anyway. They develop their pinkish hue after delving into a diet of brine shrimp and blue-green algae – food that would likely kill other animals.

Flamingos tend to live in inhospitable, relatively remote wetlands, lakes so alkaline in pH it could burn human flesh off the bones. Within this water, however, is an untapped resource of food like crustaceans, cyanobacteria and diatom algae. All of these can be dangerous to many other animals as they contain toxic chemicals called carotenoids.

69. The Pink Moon

The name itself first came to the public in the 1930s when the *Maine Farmer's Almanac* published the Native American names of the Moon for each month. Pink Moon specifically referred to the full moon in April.

That name itself is derived from the herb moss pink, one of the first flowers of spring in the eastern US.

But is the Pink Moon even pink? No. It's just a full moon called Pink Moon.

70. Approximately 70%

The truth is that an average of roughly 60%. The amount of water in the body changes slightly with age, sex, and hydration levels.

71. Backward

What may not be so well known, though, is that kangaroos cannot walk backwards. Their hopping movement is called saltation. During saltation, kangaroos push off with both large feet at the same time, and they use their tails for balance.

72. True

Yes, tiger skin is striped just like its fur. If the fur were shaved off a tiger, the skin underneath would have exactly the same markings that the fur had. The stripes serve to help conceal the tiger when its hunting or evading other prey.

73. Through their skin

They absorb water directly through their skin in an area known as the 'drinking patch' located on their belly and the underside of their thighs.

74. 6-seconds

Each of us yawns, on average, about five to 20 times a day, with each yawn lasting about five to six seconds. But why exactly do we yawn? It turns out no one knows for sure. Yawning is associated with sleepiness, but scientists haven't found that it indicates a need for sleep. It doesn't seem to be caused by the body having too little oxygen or too much carbon dioxide, which in theory could be fixed by taking a big, deep yawn.

75. Bangkok

Bangkok, Thailand's capital, is a large city known for ornate shrines and vibrant street life. The boat-filled Chao Phraya River feeds its network of canals, flowing past the Rattanakosin royal district, home to opulent Grand Palace and its sacred Wat Phra Kaew Temple.

76. About 600

The three main types of muscle include visceral, cardiac, and skeletal.
1. Visceral muscles are the weakest muscle tissues and are found inside the organs like the stomach, blood vessels, etc.

2. Cardiac muscles, as the name suggests, are found inside the heart and are responsible for pumping blood.

3. The skeletal muscles are the only voluntary muscle tissues found inside the human body. These are responsible for locomotion and movement such as speaking, walking et cetera.

77. An army

Irrespective of the species of frogs in question and whether they live in water or on land, a group is called an army because an army generally refers to a large collective.

78. A group of foxes is called a skulk

The word skulk comes from a Scandinavian word, and generally means to wait, lurk or move stealthily.

79. A banana

Many of the "housekeeping" genes that are necessary for basic cellular function, such as for replicating DNA, controlling the cell cycle, and helping cells divide are shared between many plants (including bananas) and animals." Humans share approximately 98% of their DNA with chimps, 70% with slugs, and 50% with bananas!

80. A hummingbird

The unique architecture of its wings enables it to fly forward, backward, straight up and down, or to remain suspended in the air.

81. Belgium

Common lore claims that the original fry was born in Namur in francophone Belgium, where the locals were particularly fond of fried fish. When the River Meuse froze over one cold winter in 1680, people ostensibly fried potatoes instead of the small fish they were accustomed to, and the fry was born.

82. Approximately one trillion different scents

Humans can distinguish more than 1 trillion scents, according to new research. The findings show that our sense of smell is far more discriminating than previously thought. When you stroll through a garden, you may notice several shades of golden daffodils and recognize the chirping of several types of birds.

83. Blue

The blue blood is because the protein, hemocyanin, which carries oxygen around the octopus's body, contains copper rather than iron like we have in our own hemoglobin.

84. Octopuses

An octopus's three hearts have slightly different roles. Their two peripheral hearts pump blood through the gills, where it picks up oxygen. A central heart then circulates the oxygenated blood to the rest of the body to provide energy for organs and muscles.

Octopuses have 9 brains because, in addition to the central brain, each of 8 arms has a mini brain that allows it to act independently.

85. 1889

The very first pizza delivery is attributed to Queen Margherita of Savoy in 1889. After traveling to Naples, the queen fell ill and requested authentic Italian food from the region. Royalty at that time was not expected to go out and find the best meals, so the food had to be brought to them.

86. Star and sailor

The word "astronaut" derives from the Greek words ástron, meaning "star", and nautes, meaning "sailor".

87. Venetian

Marco Polo (1254-1324) was a Venetian merchant believed to have journeyed across Asia at the height of the Mongol Empire. He first set out at age 17 with his father and uncle, traveling overland along what later became known as the Silk Road.

88. The name, hummingbird, comes from the humming noise their wings make as they beat so fast.

89. A smack

A smack is "a sharp slap or blow typically given with the palm of the hand as a rebuke or punishment." And, that's what it feels like when you suddenly get caught in a group of jellyfish. Ouch. Other collective nouns for a group of jellyfish are bloom or swarm.

90. Apes

All of the great apes, orangutans, gorillas, chimpanzees and bonobos, respond to being tickled with a remarkably human-like laugh. Dogs, meerkats, penguins and many others also seem to enjoy it. Rats giggle ultrasonically when tickled by humans but just like humans, they need to be in the right mood for it.

91. Brain, heart, blood, and our joints even our hair

Although iron is the most abundant metal in our body, traces of gold can be found in human body in several different places. If all the pure gold found in a human body whose weight is 70kg is collected, it can amount to 0.229 milligrams of gold.

92. George Washington

On April 30, 1789, George Washington, standing on the balcony of Federal Hall on Wall Street in New York, took his oath of office as the first President of the United States.

93. Henry Dunant

Henry Dunant, also known as Henri Dunant, was a Swiss humanitarian, businessman, and social activist. He was the visionary, promoter, and co-founder of the Red Cross. In 1901, he received the first Nobel Peace Prize together with Frédéric Passy. Dunant was the first Swiss Nobel laureate.

94. 1930

On July 13, 1930, France defeats Mexico 4-1 and the United States defeats Belgium 3-0 in the first-ever World Cup football matches, played simultaneously in host city Montevideo, Uruguay. The World Cup has since become the world's most watched sporting event.

95. Independence Day

On the 4th of July in 1776, the United States gained independence from Great Britain by the Continental Congress. In an almost unanimous decision, 12 of the 13 North American colonies voted for the separation from Great Britain.

96. A litter

A group of pigs is called a drift or drove. A group of young pigs is called a litter. A group of hogs is called a passel or team. A group of swine is called a sounder. A group of boars is called a singular.

97. Corgi dogs

Elizabeth II owned more than 30 corgis from her accession in 1952 until her death in 2022. She owned at least one corgi throughout the years 1933 to 2018.

98. Between four and six chukkers in a match

Chukker: Term used for a period of play in polo. Seven and a half minutes long.

99. The boiling point of water is 212 degrees Fahrenheit or 100 degrees Celsius at sea level.

That means in most places this is the temperatures of boiled water. However, as you rise above sea level water will boil at a lower temperature.

The temperature at which water boils varies based on elevation. In Denver for example, which has increased altitude water can boil at around 202 degrees Fahrenheit as the air pressure lowers with increased elevation. On Mount Everest the boiling point of water will fall between 160- and 165-degrees Fahrenheit.

100. Tendons

These are made of strong fibrous connective tissue, and they connect muscles to bone. They appear as the long thin ends of the muscles.

Tendons may also attach muscles to structures such as the eyeball. A tendon serves to move the bone or structure. A ligament is a fibrous connective tissue that attaches bone to bone, and usually serves to hold structures together and keep them stable.

Made in the USA
Coppell, TX
11 February 2023

12608967R00090